COMMUNICATION AND AWARENESS
IN A CANCER WARD

COMMUNICATION AND AWARENESS IN A CANCER WARD

JIM McINTOSH

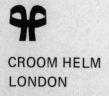

CROOM HELM
LONDON

PRODIST
NEW YORK

© 1977 Jim McIntosh

Croom Helm Ltd, 2-10 St John's Road, London SW11

ISBN 0-85664-407-2

First published in the United States by
PRODIST
a division of
Neale Watson Academic Publications, Inc.
156 Fifth Avenue, New York 10010

Library of Congress Cataloging in Publication Data

McIntosh, Jim.
    Communication and awareness in a cancer ward.

    Includes bibliographies.
    1. Cancer nursing. 2. Cancer—Psychological
aspects. 3. Medical personnel and patient.
4. Communication in medicine. I. Title.
RC266.M3   610.73'6   76-30331
ISBN 0-88202-109-5

Printed in Great Britain by Biddles Ltd, Guildford, Surrey

CONTENTS

ACKNOWLEDGEMENTS

Of the many people who have helped in this study one of the most central contributions was undoubtedly that of the medical and nursing staff of the Malignant Diseases Unit at Aberdeen Royal Infirmary, particularly Professor James F. Philip. Indeed, it was in response to an invitation from this Unit that the study originated. Not only did they provide the opportunity for carrying out the study, the staff of the Unit through their friendliness, forbearance, kindness and willingness to help and participate also contributed to making the fieldwork not just less lonely and uncomfortable than it otherwise might have been but also, in many ways, a happy and enjoyable one. My sincere thanks to all of them.

The study would not, of course, have been possible without the co-operation of the many patients who so willingly agreed to participate in it. To them I owe an incalculable debt. At a time when they must have had other pressing concerns, their willingness both to spend time talking to me and to permit me to observe their interactions with others is something for which I remain deeply grateful.

Colleagues at the Institute of Medical Sociology helped substantially at different stages of the study. I owe a particular debt of gratitude to the following: To Derek Gill, who supervised the study throughout, for his commitment, selfless devotion of time, encouragement, prodding and, not least, his incisive and always constructive comments upon the conduct of the study. To him I owe a huge debt. To Gordon Horobin, who shared the task of supervision latterly and made many valuable comments on various parts of the draft. His infinite patience and understanding played no small part in facilitating completion of the final manuscript. To Raymond Illsley, who negotiated access and was particularly influential in helping to shape the original conception of the study. He was also responsible for fostering in the Institute a spirit of co-operation and standards of academic excellence which contributed in no small measure to the present study.

My wife Jean provided encouragement and support throughout and made many helpful comments on the draft chapters. Her contribution was far greater than she realises.

I am extremely grateful to Sandra Short who typed the manuscript with her customary accuracy and patience. Elizabeth Connon and Anne Forbes also provided secretarial assistance at various stages.

I was supported during the study by a grant from the Medical Research Council.

1 DESIGN AND METHODS

This book seeks to advance our knowledge and understanding of a subject which has been a matter of concern and debate for decades, namely communication with cancer patients. It sets out to describe and explain the structure and organisation of the processes of communication between cancer patients and their doctors in one particular hospital context. In particular, it examines patients' awareness, their desire for information and efforts to obtain it, and the ways in which the medical and nursing staff managed communication with them and attempted to control the information which they received. A central feature of the study is a concern with the processual and interactional nature of the phenomena under investigation.

Cancer probably arouses more fear than any other disease being generally regarded as extremely painful and invariably incurable. For many it is synonomous with death (Wakefield, 1970). However, this fear of cancer is partially well founded as it is second only to cardiovascular disease as a cause of death. Indeed, it could be argued that the incidence of the disease is now of epidemic proportions. This, together with the public's conception of it, has meant that problems of communication associated with the disease have assumed a major significance in the work of many medical practitioners. Some of the greatest dilemmas which doctors face are associated with whether and how much to tell cancer patients about their illness.

The study arose in response to an invitation from the Malignant Diseases Unit of a Scottish Teaching Hospital to attempt to answer certain questions in which the Unit was interested. These questions related mainly to the patients, their knowledge of their illness, their desire for information about it, and the effectiveness, or appropriateness, of the staff's communication with them generally. However, it was clear from the outset that these issues could be examined satisfactorily only in the total context in which they obtained. Patients' awareness and reactions were likely to be inextricably interwoven with the ways in which the staff managed communication with them. This meant that the doctors' orientations and communication practices had also to be included in the study. The medical staff found this acceptable.

Communication with cancer patients has been the subject of protracted and controversial debate; much of the published work has centred on the question of whether the patient should be told. This literature has been reviewed at some length elsewhere (McIntosh 1974) and will therefore be referred to only briefly here. This study departs from previous approaches to the topic in several important respects. In order to ascertain whether and what the cancer sufferer would like to be told previous studies had drawn inferences from interviews with subjects who had been informed that they had cancer or with samples from the general population who did not have the disease (Aitken-Swan and Easson 1959; Kelly and Friesen 1950; Standard and Nathan 1955; Gilbertson and Wangensteen 1962; Paterson and Aitken-Swan 1954). Patients with diagnosed but undisclosed malignancy had seldom been studied. The patients in the present study had not been informed of their diagnosis by the medical staff. In addition, the ways in which patients' conceptions of their illness, and responses to it, might develop and change over time had not been previously examined. The question of what doctors tell cancer patients, and why they tell them what they do, had also been inadequately tackled. Previous attempts to examine doctors' practices of communication and the rationale behind them had concentrated upon their accounts of what they did and their reported reasons for telling or not telling (Fitts and Ravdin 1953; Oken 1961). Doctors had been asked about their views on, and practices of, telling, but this sort of data had not been backed up by observation of what they actually did. No systematic attempt had been made to examine doctors' ideologies on telling and to assess their relationship to practice. More importantly, though, the processual and contextual aspects of communication between cancer patients and their doctors, the way in which it might evolve and change either over time or in response to specific features of particular contexts or interactions — especially the actions of the participants to structure it in accordance with their own wishes — had not been examined. In short, previous approaches to the topic had been static, and often retrospective, and had not been addressed to the study of ongoing processes of interaction, decision-making and diffusion of information as these occurred in context. This was the focus of the present investigation.

The available resources dictated that the research be confined to one ward. This clearly precluded examination of questions and hypotheses which related to factors outside the ward setting or which would have involved studies of a comparative nature. However, the study did not set out to produce the definitive statement on communication with cancer patients. Rather, through its qualitative emphasis, it sought to complement larger scale quantitative approaches to the problem. Its central concern was to provide, by means of intensive investigation, an in-depth and processual account of awareness, information seeking and the management of communication in one particular locale. Nevertheless, while obtained in one ward, many of the findings are universal in their application. Although the setting is unique, the problems examined are not.

The task of the study was essentially twofold: to investigate the ways in which patients conceived of, and responded to, their illness, and to examine the structure and organisation of what was communicated to them. These two sides of the communication process were, of course, far from discrete and much of the study was concerned with the interaction between them. Investigation of what patients were told centred on the following questions: what did the doctors tell the patients and why did they tell them what they did? How, and for what reasons, might this differ in different contexts? Both philosophical and contextual factors were likely to be important in structuring what was communicated to patients. The work of Strauss *et al* (1964) had suggested that the doctors' ideologies on telling would be of paramount importance in determining the form and content of their communication. Explanation of what was communicated to patients therefore required consideration of the socially conditioned values and beliefs held by the doctors concerning what patients should be told. In addition, the context in which the communication had to be carried out would probably also exert a considerable influence on its structure and content. The literature suggested that uncertainty was likely to be one of the more important of such influences. Davis (1963) had found that uncertainty led to a restriction of what was communicated to the parents of child polio victims while Roth (1963) had noted the way in which it led to the control of information in a tuberculosis hospital. There can be no denying that with cancer the degree of uncertainty can be very great, as a brief consideration of the nature of the disease will demonstrate. Malignant disease is a process of cellular disorder whereby cells come to change some of their normal biochemical characteristics and acquire the ability to invade other tissues. Whereas normal cells are identifiable as belonging to a particular tissue and are incapable of survival away from their tissue of origin, malignant cells mutate, lose their resemblance to the normal cells in their tissue of origin and become capable of autonomous growth in distant sites. Such independent growth at distant sites is called metastasis and is one of the prime ways in which cancer can harm or destroy a host. Like a benign tumour, a malignant growth has escaped the growth regulating influences of the body but, unlike the benign tumour, which is circumscribed by surrounding tissues, the malignant neoplasm can infiltrate and implant itself in other parts of the body. This gives rise to two diagnostic problems for the doctor: firstly, is the tumour benign or malignant, and, secondly, has it spread? Uncertainty usually arises either because the diagnosis has not been fully established or because it is unclear what course the disease will follow in a particular case. Although there may be little doubt about the diagnosis of established cancer, the diagnosis of cancer in its early stages, and in certain sites, can be difficult and uncertain. Usually it requires a biopsy to establish that the growth is malignant. It is best to conceive of cancer, not as one disease, but rather as a group of diseases which are similar insofar as they are all malignant but which may differ quite markedly in terms of severity and outcome. Even the same categories of growth may contain examples with very different degrees of malignancy. Thus, although the outcome of some types of cancer is more easy to assess than others, the prognosis for the condition is often extremely difficult to predict with certainty. Clearly, then, uncertainty over diagnosis and outcome is likely to be a central theme in the treatment of cancer patients.

In the present context, the question was: how did the doctors manage this uncertainty in terms of what they communicated to patients? Given that the doctor might withhold information when uncertain so as to avoid subsequently being proved wrong, it would appear reasonable to suppose that once he was certain, and this restriction had been removed, he would be more willing to tell the patient about his condition. However, Davis' work (1963) suggested that the picture might not be quite as simple as that. He found that, in the case of child polio victims, even when certain of the prognosis, the doctors did not pass on the information to parents. This led him to develop a distinction between clinical and functional uncertainty (1966). Clinical uncertainty is based upon real difficulties in diagnosis and prognosis whereas functional uncertainty exists after clinical certainty has been established and serves to aid the doctor in the management of patients. Davis demonstrates how, 'uncertainty, a real factor in the early diagnosis and treatment of the paralysed child, came more and more to serve the purely managerial ends of the treatment personnel in their interaction with parents', (1966, 316). That is, *professions* of uncertainty were used to limit what was disclosed. If the cancer patients were not informed about their condition once the diagnosis and prognosis had been established, the withholding of information had clearly to be explained in terms of factors other than the management of clinical uncertainty.

Some doctors argue that what patients are told depends upon their perception of individual patients and their circumstances.[1] However, if the doctors in the present study based their communication upon the assessment of individuals, they were likely to have to contend with other types of uncertainty. They would probably be uncertain of how much the patient wanted to know and how he was likely to react to disclosure. The ways in which they managed or resolved these uncertainties would clearly be important in determining what the patient was told. It was also possible that, faced with these uncertainties, the doctor might base his decisions on what to tell patients upon certain assumptions which he made about them (Freidson 1970, p. 142). Previous work on uncertainty (Scheff 1963, Roth 1958) suggested that one of the ways in which it might be managed was through the adoption of informal norms and the routinization of procedures. These procedures were, moreover, likely to be based upon typifications of patients and conditions (Scheff 1968, Sudnow 1968). It was therefore hypothesized that, in the event of uncertainty, communication would be based upon typifications of patients and conditions and that each typification would have ascribed to it an appropriate course of action.

The following questions were formulated in relation to the patients. How much did they know about their condition? How did their awareness change over the course of their stay in hospital and what factors contributed to this? How much did the patients want to know? How did they attempt to obtain information? How much did they find out and from what sources? Why might some patients not want to know? Again uncertainty was likely to be an important feature, especially if the patients were not formally given their diagnosis and prognosis. How might they cope with it? Roth (1963) had demonstrated that one of the ways in which patients attempt to reduce or eradicate uncertainty is by seeking information about their condition. However, if the staff did not want to disclose to the patients, their quest for information was likely to prove a difficult exercise. In that event, the patients might resort to certain tactics to obtain the information they wanted. Roth (1963) had described the way in which TB patients bargained for information about their condition while some of the more subterranean methods by which dying patients sought to find out about their illness had been documented by Glaser and Strauss (1965, pp. 53-55). Alternatively, it was possible that, as a consequence of difficulty in obtaining information through official channels, inquisitive patients might turn to informal sources for the information which they sought. Informal sources of information might therefore constitute an important component in the total process of communication and information seeking. Most of the data sought on the informal network was of a descriptive nature and related to one central hypothesis. It was that 'restriction of formal communication to patients, and a lack of success in information seeking within the formal channels, will lead them to seek information within the informal network'. There were likely to be a number of possible informal sources of information. Firstly, information might be obtained informally from a number of non-medical personnel, with whom the patient would be in contact while in hospital. These might include, physiotherapists, radiographers, social workers, cleaners, porters and the clergy. Even nurses, although officially instructed not to do so, might, either deliberately or inadvertently, pass information on to patients. Investigation of the role of the nurse in the total communication process was to be an important aspect of the study. How much were they permitted to convey to patients and how did they manage communication with them? In addition to information conveyed to them informally by word of mouth, a number of clues, such as the type of treatment which they received, were also likely to be available to patients who sought to find out about their condition (Glaser and Strauss 1965; Hinton 1967, pp. 98-99; Kelly and Friesen 1950, p. 822; Verwoerdt 1966, p. 17). Fellow patients were another possible source of information. Roth (1963) had shown that one of the ways in which patients attempt to find out about their condition is by comparing themselves with others whom they perceive as having a condition which does, or did, approximate their own. The fact that patients discuss their conditions with each other and exchange information had also been well documented (Cartwright 1964; Roth in Freidson 1963; Davis 1963). However, none of the above authors were studying cancer patients and Glaser and Strauss (1965), in their study of dying, found that on a cancer ward the rules of 'tact' were so strong that few patients talked openly about anyone's condition. There was also some evidence that hospital patients, sharing a common situation, might form groups in order to work out solutions to their mutual problems (Caudill 1958; Stanton and Schwartz 1954) and it was decided to attempt to establish the extent to which this was so with the patients to be studied.

While examination of the ways in which patients sought to obtain information was clearly important, the converse might also require explanation. Some patients might *not* seek to find out about their condition. Apart from a reluctance to question due to diffidence (Cartwright 1964), a wish not to appear a nuisance (Freidson 1961), a desire not to expose their ignorance of medical matters (Cartwright 1964), the perceived social distance between themselves and the doctor (Skipper 1965) or the strategies of information control employed by the staff (Freidson 1961, p. 51), they might quite simply not want to know. Investigation into the reasons for patients not wanting to know was to form an important part of the study. Another important question, given the number of clues which were likely to be present, was how did patients who did not want to know avoid becoming aware of the nature of their condition? While denial by cancer patients that they had the disease had been recorded (Kubler-Ross 1969, pp. 34-43), even among patients who had been explicitly told (Rothenberg 1961), the ways in which they avoided realization had not been so closely examined.

An examination of the processes of communication would not have been complete had it not considered what was communicated to relatives and the role which they played in the total communication network. The central questions here were: what were relatives told and did they pass information on to the patients? It appeared that relatives of cancer patients were much more likely to be informed about the patient's condition than the patient himself (Quint 1964; Oken 1961). However, why this should be so was unclear. The fact that collusion occurred between doctors and relatives in withholding information from the patient had also been well documented (Glaser and Strauss 1965; Quint 1964). But, whether relatives withheld information because they were persuaded to do so by the doctor or whether it was because they simply shared his perspectives, was a matter for further study.

Each of the questions and hypotheses set out above required the collection of data on the behaviour and perceptions of at least one of the following: patients, doctors, nurses, relatives and other hospital workers. Frequently, the information required did not relate to the behaviour and perceptions of one individual or group but to an interaction over time between pairs or more. For example, data on the doctors' beliefs about telling could be obtained simply through interviewing the doctors, whereas information on how the patients coped with uncertainty required, as a minimum, interviews with the patients and observation of staff-patient interactions. If the patients' management of uncertainty involved information seeking within the informal network, then information on their interactions with fellow patients, relatives and other hospital personnel had to be obtained. The next section discusses the ways in which these proposals were implemented.

Methodology

The study was conducted by means of a combination of observation and interviewing. A detailed description of what transpired on the ward, and examination of the processual and interactional nature of the phenomena, required direct observation of the processes under investigation (Becker and Geer 1957). Two types of question were involved: one descriptive, the other explanatory. While documentation of what occurred on the ward could be obtained by means of careful and comprehensive observation, explanation of the observed processes could only be achieved through an analysis of comparative observations. However, certain data could not be obtained through observation. Accordingly, in order to assess patients' knowledge of their illness, desire for information about it and how these might change over the course of hospitalization, 80 patients (52 women and 28 men) were interviewed formally upon admission and, again, on discharge. Similarly, members of the medical and nursing staff were interviewed to obtain their views on communicating with cancer patients. The two methods were differentially appropriate for obtaining different sorts of information. They were complementary and equally essential (Stacey 1969, p. 67; McCall and Simmons 1969, pp. 4-5). In addition, though, each method, in part, provided a check on the validity of the data being obtained by the other (Denzin 1970). While the formal interviewing programme was accomplished in six months, altogether one year was spent observing interactions on the ward.

Ward 4C was not entirely occupied by cancer patients. They shared the ward with dental and gynaecology patients. There were eight beds for cancer patients in the female ward while, at the male end, there were ten beds in the main ward and one bed in a side ward for men and a two-bed side ward for women. Therefore, the total number of cancer patients who could be in the ward at any one time was twenty one. The remainder of the beds were occupied by a gynaecology overspill from another ward in the female end and dental patients in the male ward. The cancer patients occupied the beds nearest to the entrance in both wards while the others were allocated beds at the far end of the ward and in the balconies. Thus, the distinct groups in terms of diagnosis were grouped together physically. The length of stay for the cancer patients was highly variable: some were in for two nights and others for many weeks. The turnover among the women was almost twice as rapid as among the men giving an admission ratio of five females for every three males.

The range of conditions treated on the ward was so great that an attempt to make comparisons by type of condition would have required a much larger sample than would have been compatible with the intensive nature of the study and the time available. In order to eliminate sampling bias it was proposed that the interview sample should consist of all cases admitted to the ward over a specified period. However, in practice it was not possible to include all patients in the study: some were too old and confused, others were deaf and still others were too ill to interview. Only two patients declined to take part. No other grounds were used for excluding patients from the sample. While the most common types of cancer treated on the ward were those of the breast, skin and head and neck, a wide range of conditions was represented. Some were primary lesions while others were recurrences or secondary deposits of the disease. So the sample encompassed a considerable variety of conditions in terms of location, severity, and extent of involvement of the disease.

The observation technique consisted of observing as much as possible of the interaction which occurred between various groups and individuals in different contexts, recording what was said by whom and to whom and, in this way, gradually building up a picture of the processes being examined. Such extensive observation allowed for the emergence of fresh insights and the generation of new hypotheses. These data were supplemented by a series of relatively casual interviews, or chats, which were conducted with the subjects throughout the study. For example, part of the observation method involved talking to the patients, at intervals, about their perceptions of their condition and progress, their desire for additional information and their degree of success in obtaining it. This, together with the more formal interviews, enabled the monitoring of development and change in patients' conceptions of their illness, and responses to it, and the identification of causal factors. In addition to observing on the ward, I also observed interaction in the ward precincts, attended the weekly conferences and spent a period in the outpatient department.

Between the extremes of pure participant and non-participant observation there is a continuum of observation techniques defined by varying degrees of involvement with subjects and immersement in their experiences (Stacey 1969, pp. 50-68; Cicourel 1964, pp. 43-45; Gold 1958). Clearly, I could not engage in total participant observation with any of the subjects as this would have required, in turn, being admitted as a patient, working as a nurse and being employed on the ward as a doctor. What I attempted to do, therefore, was to become as closely involved in the lives of the subjects as was possible, given the constraints just mentioned. I tried to get as near as I could to acceptance as a member of their particular group. The degree of participation involved varied at different times and in different settings. For example, I would often become involved in doctors' conversations but only observe their interaction with patients. Similarly with patients, I would on occasion take part in their conversations while at other times I would simply observe the discussion.

However, observation was not without its difficulties. A particular problem at the beginning of the study was that of where to position myself in order to observe the interaction, particularly that which occurred among the patients. If I stationed myself at any particular point in the ward, I found that I could observe who talked to whom but could hear little of what was being said. Clearly, taking up fixed positions in the ward was not going to be very productive in terms of data collection. In an attempt to overcome this, I tried wandering through the ward in an effort to eavesdrop on conversations by stopping in the vicinity of patient interactions—either reading or writing in my notebook—to see if anything relevant to my interests was being discussed. This method yielded little and was anyway one about which I had grave reservations. Although the patients had been informed that I was conducting a study on the ward and had not objected to my presence, I did not want to seem, or rather to be seen, to be eavesdropping. That might appear rude. And, for obvious reasons, I wanted the patients to think well of me.

These attempts at observation were also accompanied by a sense of extreme conspicuousness and an associated feeling of great discomfort. I was very conscious of the fact that I probably appeared slightly odd to the patients, hanging about the ward with no apparent duties apart from looking around me and occasionally jotting something in my notebook.[2] I attempted to alleviate this by trying to appear busy, often by pretending to write in my notebook, but, even then, 30-45 minutes in observation was as much as I could stand.

My initial attempts at observation were, then, largely unsuccessful and accompanied by considerable discomfort. Clearly, I could not observe effectively as a detached onlooker. A compromise solution had to be found and, fortunately, was. What I did was to circulate patient groupings and, as far as I could, join in their conversations as if I was one of them. In other words, I attempted, as far as was possible, to enter into their world, to take part in their discussions, and to gain acceptance as an, admittedly marginal, member of their group. This was largely successful but not without its difficulties. At first, patients were a little chary, and perhaps somewhat bemused, at my presence. For example, if I joined an ongoing conversation it tended to stop in midstream with the patients looking at me wondering what I wanted. I was not yet expected to drop in on conversations. I got round this by saying, 'Carry on. I have a bit of time to kill so I thought I'd join you for a while.' They usually carried on. However, in time, once I had become more familiar to them and they had come to trust me, they accepted my presence quite naturally and came to discuss their illnesses quite freely in my company. Sometimes a conversation which I had joined would drift on to the theme of illness. On other occasions I would subtly introduce the topic by asking a patient how he or she was getting on, how the operation went, or some other general question about treatment or progress. Invariably, the rest of the group would join in, adding their comments and relating their own experiences and fears. Many of these discussions might not have taken place but for my intervention. However, I was interested in their content not their frequency of occurrence. I wanted to observe how patients discussed their illnesses—if at all—the terms which they used and the way in which they presented their condition to their fellow patients. These observational data on patient interactions were supplemented by questioning patients about them in the interviews.

I did not face these difficulties in observing interactions among the medical and nursing staff. With them I was much more of a participant observer — not in the sense that I shared in the treatment of patients but because they came to view me as one of the group. I had no problems of being excluded from interactions and, as far as I was aware, the doctors did not avoid discussing certain topics in my presence. Indeed, I was privy to conversations which would have caused considerable embarrassment if they had been repeated by me.

Fortunately, too, observation of doctor-patient interactions was relatively straightforward and unproblematic. I could easily attach myself to the doctors on a ward round or when they went to see a particular patient. One difficulty which I did experience while accompanying the doctors was in hearing what was being said behind the screens while patients were being examined. It had been decided that, for ethical reasons, I should not attend the examination of patients. For the majority of examinations I was able to hear clearly but there were occasions on which the voices were too low for me to hear properly or when I missed parts of a conversation. In that event, I asked the doctors about what had transpired.

Nurse-patient interaction was much more difficult to observe. While it was possible to observe doctor-patient encounters in a fairly comprehensive way, this was not so with the nurses. The principal problem was the sheer volume of such interaction. The nurses were working on the ward, and therefore interacting with the patients, almost continuously. Moreover, several nurse-patient encounters were usually ongoing at any particular point in time. Much of the interaction was therefore inevitably missed. In addition, the problem of observing the nurses' management of communication with patients was compounded by the elusiveness of nurse-patient interactions in which the nature and severity of the patient's illness was raised. Discussion of this topic was relatively infrequent and, also, probably less likely to occur in my presence. My observations of such encounters were therefore limited in number. Nevertheless, those which were observed did yield sufficient data, in conjunction with other sources of information, to enable certain conclusions about the nature of nurse-patient communication to be drawn.

For recording my observations I used pocket-size shorthand notebooks and dated all entries. I seldom recorded material on the spot apart from in ward conferences, in the outpatient clinic, and while engaged in general observation on the ward. I decided not to take notes while observing interactions between the various participants or while in the company of patients. There were two reasons for this. Firstly, notetaking would have entailed a shift in my attention from what I wanted to observe and, secondly, might have made the subjects feel uncomfortable and behave atypically (McCall and Simmons 1969, p. 73). Instead, during observation, I memorised key phrases, or a few words, which would summarise a conversation or interaction. I found little difficulty in recall if I used this method and recorded the observations as soon as possible when I got a quiet moment in the resident's room. If I had to wait longer before putting the data into my notebook, I would always endeavour to get the key words or phrases written down. As there were a limited number of significant verbal exchanges during any period of observation or ward round, often only two or three, I found it relatively easy to record these verbatim from memory. I would also mentally relive a ward round or period of observation to see if I had omitted anything. In this way, I occasionally recalled something that I had forgotten.

Something which I experienced quite strongly during the study was a feeling of marginality. This was unpleasant rather than of any practical significance for the conduct of the research. Much of the discomfort which I have described experiencing during observation was, of course, in part a product of this perception of the marginality of my role. There were two related senses in which I felt peripheral. I felt, firstly, that I did not belong, that I was an outsider, and, secondly, that I had no useful task to perform. 'Everyone but me seems to be part of a team, a cohesive unit, each member of which has a clearly defined role and is working towards a specific end, namely the treatment and care of patients. I am neither a member of that team nor are our goals the same.' (Fieldnotes June 3, 1971.)

As I was in no way able to contribute to the work of the Unit, I worried about whether I was regarded as a nuisance simply following people around and watching them at work. I felt wholly parasitic. After some contact with the disease, I also came to feel that my work was less important, and the rewards less immediate, than that of the staff. 'Sometimes I feel that my work pales into insignificance alongside that of the medical staff. They are engaged in fighting the disease and I would love to be able to help.' (Fieldnotes, June 12, 1971.)

However, these matters partly resolved themselves in time as I got to know the staff better on a personal level and became accepted into their group and as they expressed continued interest in the study and assured me of its relevance to their work.

It did, however, take me a little while to gain the confidence of the nurses. I had assumed that, having informed the Sisters, an account of what I was doing would filter through to them. This was a miscalculation. One staff nurse thought that I was there to take over part of their job and when I asked a question of another nurse she expressed concern that what she said might be taken down and used against her. Two other nurses asked, 'What exactly *are* you doing?' Clearly, the nurses had not been informed of my function on the ward and, thereafter, I was careful to explain to them what I was studying.

The interviews with members of staff presented no problems. They were tape-recorded with their agreement. Those with the patients were also relatively unproblematic. They were interviewed in a side ward, when it was vacant, or at the bedside with the screens drawn. I recorded the interviews with the patients by hand, on the interview schedule, as it was felt that they might find a tape-recorder threatening and inhibiting. Although this method of recording did, at times, break the flow of the interview, overall it was quite satisfactory. What problems, or potential problems, there were in interviewing the patients related primarily to the sensitive nature of the topic under investigation. This posed problems in relation to the way in which the study should be presented to them. On ethical grounds, patients should be told exactly what a study, in which they are asked to participate, is about. Clearly, however, it was not possible to tell the patients that the focus of the present study was cancer. Instead, it was presented to them as being primarily con-

cerned with communication. The patients were therefore told the truth
about the study as explicitly as was possible without mentioning
cancer. In addition, having been informed that communication practices were the focus of the investigation, questions about what they
knew, what they had been told, whether they were satisfied with that
and what else they would like to know, appeared perfectly natural to
them in the context of the study as it had been presented to them and,
as far as could be ascertained, aroused no suspicion.

The nature of the subject matter did, of course, also make the conduct of the interviews potentially tricky. But, perhaps surprisingly, any
fears which I had along these lines proved to be largely unfounded. Certainly I was very apprehensive initially about how the interviews would
go. I was frightened in case I inadvertently let something slip or responded inadequately to patients' questions. Fortunately, I did not get involved in any tricky discussions with them. Nor did patients questioning
me about their illness present any problem. They seldom asked me anything about their condition or treatment but, if they did, I simply plead-
ed ignorance. Mostly, the patients were sufficiently aware of my role to
see me as not being an appropriate source of information. I reinforced
this by yielding none. It is difficult to say how the patients defined me
other than as a researcher and someone who asked them a lot of questions. Nor did they seem concerned to find out in greater detail who I
was or what I was doing. Doubtless, different patients defined me differently but this was probably not significant. They probably had a
tendency to identify me with the hospital staff, especially as I accompanied the doctors on their rounds, but I tried to impress upon them that
I was an independent worker in no way connected with the hospital. I
wore a white coat, for hygienic purposes, while on the ward, and
explained to patients that this was my only reason for doing so. On the
coat I wore a badge which proclaimed my identity as 'J. McIntosh,
Sociologist'. I had no reason to suspect that the patients' definitions of
me inhibited them in interviews.

Nor was I aware of any observer-effect during the study although I
cannot honestly be sure that none existed. In doctor-patient interactions
I was very much a peripheral figure, seen as such by the parties involved and hence probably not sufficiently significant to affect the content
of discussions which were, to the participants, much more important
than my presence. In other words, most of the time, I was forgotten.
The doctors and nurses would not, I believe, have been able to keep up
a consistent pretence for the duration of fieldwork. I got round the fact
that my very presence on the ward might suggest its atypicality to pat-

ients by telling them that the reason I was doing the study in that particular ward was because the head of my department knew one of the consultants there. The staff were not given any feedback, either on individual patients or my conclusions in general, during the study.

Observer bias is another matter and I must confess that at the beginning of the study I was biased to the view that patients should be given their diagnosis. I believed, firstly, that they had a right to be told and, secondly, that they would probably react well to being informed. In this I had been influenced by some of the literature on the subject which tended to suggest that cancer patients reacted better to being openly informed about their condition than to being kept in the dark. However, very soon I came to realise that my original notion of what the proper procedure for communicating with cancer patients should be predicated too simplistic an approach to the problem. The whole question was more complex than I had imagined. For example, many patients did not want to know. With this humbling realization, my impartiality as an observer was thereafter assured.

The interviews with the patients were semi-structured. They were structured insofar as there were certain areas which I wished to tap and specific questions which I wanted to ask. However, they were flexible in that I followed up any leads which emerged and made use of any opportunity for discussing cancer in greater depth with the patient. The degree to which patients were prepared to talk about their illness varied considerably. As it was, though, the great majority of patients themselves mentioned cancer and, once the term had been introduced by them, I could question them more openly on their feelings about the disease. But I still had to tread warily. I never divulged to them that the major focus of the study was cancer nor could I question them too closely about the disease itself because, again, ostensibly, it was not the main focus of the investigation. During an interview patients would sometimes indicate to me that I could pursue a particular line of questioning so far and no further, either because they did not wish to respond in greater depth or because I sensed that to do so would cause them distress. I must add, though, that this occurred rather infrequently. Often this sort of communication was transmitted and perceived at the subliminal level.[3] Communication on this level is no doubt a feature of all interactions. However, it is likely to assume particular significance in unstructured or open-ended interviews, especially where the topic of investigation is a sensitive one. In such situations the interviewer is probably constantly on the alert for, and responding to, cues which indicate how the subject is reacting to a particular line of enquiry and how he is likely to receive other questions.

One problem which I had not anticipated in relation to interviewing the patients was associated with how fully their time in the hospital was occupied. Radiotherapy, X-rays, operations, meals, visiting times, dressings, afternoon naps and doctors' rounds all intervened. Often I had to seek an interview with them on several occasions before being successful. Even then an interview might have to be interrupted and resumed later. These were minor irritations, however, and no interviews were missed because of them.

It is probably misleading to talk of stages in fieldwork, although it does follow a rough pattern (Strauss *et al* 1964, pp. 19-21), because all the time one is simultaneously deriving and testing hypotheses, collecting data, analysing and writing up. Much of my fieldwork was concerned with the testing, modification and refinement of the concepts and hypotheses presented earlier in the chapter. However, consistent with a grounded theory approach (Glaser and Strauss 1967), changes in emphasis and focus and the derivation and reformulation of hypotheses occurred throughout fieldwork. The analytic induction method was used for analysing the material (Cressey in Robinson 1969). By this method, if the individual hypothesis held for all the cases observed, this was taken as objective validation of it. If all the cases did not fit the hypothesis then alternative hypotheses were formulated until all cases were accommodated.

At the end of fieldwork I had twelve notebooks containing a record of my experiences, informal interviews and chats with patients, doctors, nurses and auxillary staff, and observations of every permutation of interactions between these groups, in many different contexts. I had formal interview data on eighty patients plus a record of observations and informal interviews with many others. I interviewed seven of the medical staff, four consultants, one senior house officer and two residents, and ten of the nursing staff, two sisters, three staff nurses and five student nurses. In addition, I had observation and informal interview data on another two residents, one senior house officer, three consultants and many more nurses. These additional informants were not interviewed formally, either because they had left the ward by the end of the study, or, as in the case of the three consultants, only occasionally attended the ward in a consultative capacity. I also interviewed the medical social worker attached to the ward. Unfortunately, my resources were such that I was unable to interview relatives and, apart from observation of a handful of doctor-relative encounters, I had to rely upon information obtained from patients, doctors, nurses and the medical social worker for information on them. The rest of the book reports on what the analysis of these data revealed.

Notes

1. However, the avowed policy of many doctors of treating each case on its merits does not appear to be reflected in practice, with the great majority either telling or not telling all their patients (Glaser and Strauss 1965, pp. 119-120). Most seem to adopt a policy of not telling (Fitts and Ravdin 1953, Oken 1961).
2. I should point out that these feelings were all purely subjective in origin and that none of the patients, as far as I was aware, had commented upon my presence in a derogatory or puzzled fashion although some had asked the nurses about me and were told that I was 'some sort of researcher'.
3. The importance of subliminal cues in an interview has been stressed by Goode and Hatt (1952).

2 THE MANAGEMENT OF UNCERTAINTY

The next three chapters are concerned with analysis and description of the methods of communication employed by the doctors on Ward 4C. The questions to be addressed are: what did the doctors tell the patients; why did they tell them what they did; and how, and for what reasons, did this differ in different contexts? These communication practices are conceived of, and analysed, in terms of the management of uncertainty.

Philosophy on Telling

All the doctors on the ward under investigation firmly believed that the great majority of patients should not be told that they had cancer or be given their prognosis unless, of course, in the case of the latter, their condition was eminently curable. Patients were to be given as much information as possible about their condition and treatment short of divulging the precise nature of the illness and consistent with their retention of hope. This policy was endorsed by all the doctors on the ward. Indeed, this also appeared to be the universal ideological standpoint on what the cancer patient should be told throughout the hospital.[1] The doctors' conviction was largely founded upon certain assumptions which they made about patients' desire for information and probable reactions to disclosure. They assumed that patients did not want to know and would react badly to being told.

> I'm sure the vast majority of patients don't want to be told what they've got. And, if we were to tell them, most of them would take it very badly I'm quite sure. Some would just go to pieces completely.[2]

Even if patients asked directly their enquiries were assumed to be requests for reassurance and not genuine attempts to find out the truth. 'Some people will ask. Now you *know* that they are asking because they want to be told that it is not.'

Associated with this was a very genuine concern for patient welfare. While aware that reactions would differ enormously and while accepting that some patients might react well to disclosure, the doctors anticipated that informing patients that they had cancer would have certain adverse and traumatic effects upon the majority of them. They believed that most patients who were told would become extremely anxious and depressed (even mentally unstable), and might withdraw completely and simply await death. This belief was based, in part, upon a limited experience of patients who had been informed of the nature of their condition.

The people we get from America who come back to this country to die, or to visit relatives before they're dead, they're like zombies. They might come in here with a relative and just sit and hardly say a word. He's been told he's only got six months to live, you see. And, right enough, they're probably right in the facts. But the patient is as important as the lump, and the relatives have to live with the patient and the patient's got to live with the relatives and it's much better somebody taking part in family life than sitting miserably in the corner waiting for the undertaker. I remember one young lad who came here from Rhodesia. It was pathetic. He was lying in a bed that looked like a bier in the middle of the floor. He had been told in Rhodesia that he had three months to live and his three months were going to be up in ten days time, and he was just lying waiting for it. I tried to instil some measure of confidence in him, although his condition was hopeless, and got him into hospital. He cheered up and was bright and reading the newspapers and his deadline passed. He lasted a few weeks but the disease got beyond us. But there was some kind of response, and the temporary change in that man's attitude towards the people surrounding him and looking after him, and his family, was well worth the effort. So, these are the things that people who tell patients that they've got cancer lose.

Above all, though, it was anticipated that patients who were informed that they had cancer would lose all hope. Leaving patients with hope of recovery was one of the main concerns of the medical staff. 'I think the basic rule applies . . . to give the patient first of all encouragement, to give hope, to make them feel it isn't the end of the world.'

The doctors similarly believed that to have revealed an unfavourable prognosis to patients would have had a shattering effect upon most of them. However, there was an added complication where the prognosis was concerned. While the doctors could usually be certain of the diagnosis often they could not be at all sure of the outlook. They could all relate tales of having been mistaken in their assessment of the course and duration of particular examples of the illness and even, occasionally, in their judgement of the final outcome. Thus, any assessment of the prognosis which was hazarded would often have amounted to little more than informed speculation. This added to their reluctance to communicate such information to patients.

In addition, of course, a negative reaction from patients could also make life more difficult for the doctors. They were all agreed that patients who were aware of what they had would, by and large, be more difficult to manage. Some might withdraw and become impossible to interact with while others might refuse to continue with treatment. Still others might react to fear and depression by involving the doctors in lengthy and complex discussions about the nature of their illness thereby obliging them 'to spend an awful lot of time with them giving them some degree of confidence and reassurance'. All this could be very time-consuming and taxing for the doctor. Moreover, if patients were aware that they had cancer, the doctors would lose much of their control over the way in which they conceived of their illness. The doctors' reluctance to disclose, and associated concern over patients' probable reactions to the knowledge that they had a malignancy, was largely based upon their perception of the way in which the general public regarded the disease. Most people, they believed, thought cancer to be incurable—'I think that the general public's idea of cancer is that once you have cancer you're finished, you're dead. There's no treatment for cancer.' Upon disclosure, these lay conceptions of the disease would come to dominate the ways in which patients conceived of their condition making it much more difficult for the doctor to instil in them an optimistic orientation towards their illness. In short, then, the doctors believed that disclosing to patients would mean trouble for all concerned.

However, while asserting that most patients did not want to know, the doctors also simultaneously held the view that many of them were aware that they had cancer. How could these two seemingly conflicting beliefs co-exist? The resolution of this apparent paradox hinges upon the premise that patients could not be absolutely certain that they had the disease in the absence of official confirmation. What the doctors actually meant when expressing the view that many patients knew what they had was that a large number strongly *suspected* that they had cancer. Otherwise, their endeavours to disclaim or conceal this fact would have been futile. Again the element of hope was present the belief being that, although patients might have had a strong suspicion that they had cancer, they could still retain hope so long as this had not been confirmed by the medical staff.

Well, speaking very broadly, I don't think in fact I know that the majority of patients do not want to be told outright what they have got. But I am sure they know. I think the fact that they are not told outright gives them some degree of comfort and solace in the long watches of the night. If they suspect, they can console themselves with the thought, 'Oh well, they didn't actually say it was cancer—it might not be'.

The belief that many patients had a quite highly developed awareness or suspicion of the nature of their condition was therefore wholly consistent with the view that they did not wish to be told outright.

Had the doctors believed that no patients should be told, their course of action would have been relatively unproblematic. However, the doctors' philosophy on telling did not wholly exclude informing patients of their diagnosis or, indeed, giving them an assessment of the outlook for their condition. While of the opinion that patients in general did not want to be told, the doctors also acknowledged that some patients would genuinely want to know and expressed the view that, where they could be counted upon not to react unfavourably, they should be informed. This was where the problem arose. The dichotomous nature of their philosophy introduced an element of choice and decision-making into what they communicated to patients. Translating this philosophical position into action was not a straightforward matter. Its implementation had to take account of a number of attendant uncertainties.

Uncertainty

As outlined in the first chapter, an important feature of neoplastic disease is the uncertainty which commonly attends it. Part of the uncertainty associated with malignancy is purely clinical: doctors usually cannot be certain the disease is cancer until investigations, usually a biopsy, have been carried out while the outcome of the illness can often be notoriously difficult to predict. Following Davis (1963, 1966) it was hypothesised that this uncertainty, and the way in which it was managed, was likely to play a major part in structuring the form and content of communication about the disease. However, clinical uncertainty was not found to be a central determinant of what was or was not communicated to patients except in cases where the doctor intended to inform them. Only in the case of benign conditions or eminently curable cancers, where the doctor intended to tell, could uncertainty over the clinical details of the case restrict what the patient was told. With these conditions, the doctors were very positive in their belief that patients should be informed that their condition was harmless or that they

were cured. However, as the doctor would not implement his intention
to tell until the diagnosis or prognosis had been established conclusively,
clinical uncertainty could, at certain stages, delay the rendering of a
favourable account of the patient's condition. When the doctors were
sure of their ground, patients were left in no doubt about the non-
serious nature of their complaint although, even then, no reference was
made to cancer. 'It was all clear—completely benign—nothing to worry
about.'

'We took this out. It was just a simple thing. (Cancer) It'll give you
no more bother.'

But, while they intended to tell where the condition was benign or
where the malignancy had clearly been eradicated, with all other
examples of the disease the doctors had no such intention. In the case
of the latter, even when certain of the diagnosis and prognosis, they
would not disclose them to patients. Clearly, then, factors other than
clinical uncertainty were responsible for the withholding of information
from these patients. This concurs with Davis's work (1966) on child
polio victims where he found that, even after clinical certainty had been
established, doctors did not pass the information on to parents and
instead continued to profess to be uncertain of the child's prognosis.
He concludes that 'clearly . . . clinical uncertainty is not responsible
for all that is not communicated to the patient and his family. Other
factors, interests and circumstances intrude in the rendering of medical
prognoses . . .' (p. 318). In the present context, the withholding of
information from patients is best explained in terms of the ways in
which the doctors coped with other forms of uncertainty. These uncertainties are associated with patients' desire for information and probable reactions to disclosure. Quite simply, while the doctors accepted
that some patients would genuinely want to know and would not react
adversely, they did not know *which* patients really wanted to know or
which of them would react well to being told. Nor was there any way
in which these uncertainties could be resolved. There was no way of
gauging accurately what patients' desire for information and possible
reactions to disclosure were. Even a patient who asked outright might
simply be seeking reassurance. To be sure, the doctors had theories
about the kind of patient who might 'really' want to know and who
would react well to being told, for example, patients with family or
business commitments or the professional as opposed to other classes.
However, these did not provide a sufficiently accurate basis on which
to make decisions. The doctor could not proceed on the basis of general-
ities, which were based upon assumptions, when deciding whether or

not to disclose. For that exercise he would require precise information on individual patients. In short then, there was no certain basis on which to make decisions on whether or not to tell particular patients. Some measure of uncertainty was always present. Because this uncertainty could not be resolved it had somehow to be managed. How was this achieved in terms of what was communicated to patients?

There were two ways in which the doctors coped with these uncertainties consistent with their view that the great majority of patients did not want to know and would react badly to being told, and their overriding concern to leave patients with hope. Firstly, they adopted the only safe course of action open to them: they did not disclose to any of the patients unless it was absolutely necessary to do so. This response was informed by the general principle that not to tell a patient who did want to know was to be preferred to telling a patient who did not want to know and who might react badly to disclosure.[3] In this way, the risk of informing someone who either did not want to know or who could not take the news was eliminated. Communication was characterized by avoidance of the terms 'cancer' and 'malignancy'. The more serious aspects and ramifications of the patient's condition were also played down or not explicitly referred to. However, this should not be taken to imply that the patients were lied to. They were not.[4] Certain information was simply withheld from them. Communication was conducted by means of euphemisms which, while comprising the truth, (for example, a patient's tumour could quite legitimately be said to contain some 'nasty cells') stopped short of full disclosure. The euphemistic content of their communication enabled the doctors to avoid giving explicit information while, at the same time, not telling any lies. What patients were told was not untrue, it was simply not the whole truth. Secondly, all communication to patients was routinized.[5] The routinisation of communication provided ways of managing uncertainty in accordance with the doctors' beliefs about patients' desire for information and probable reactions to being told. The routines were geared to limiting the amount of disclosure to patients. There were routine procedures pertaining to what was volunteered to patients and a separate set of routine responses to specific types of patient demand. These routines were differentially appropriate for different categories of condition, in terms of severity, at different stages of their treatment. In other words, telling was based upon typifications of cases.[6] Thus, what was volunteered to a patient depended upon the category to which his condition belonged not upon his individual case. Similarly, what patients were told in response to enquiries depended upon the routine

responses appropriate to particular questions, posed by people with
particular types of condition, not upon assessment of their particular
circumstances.

The observation that communication was routinized to a large
extent conflicted with the doctors' own perceptions of their communication practices. They maintained that what was communicated to patients, and whether or not they disclosed to them, depended upon their
assessment of each individual case.

> I think you have to treat everyone as an individual. You must get to
> know your patient well so that you have a sort of insight into how
> much a patient can stand. What does he want to know? Does he want
> to know he's got cancer? Does he want to know how long he's got to
> live? Does he want to know what his chances are? You've got to
> make your mind up about this.

> I think that each patient is dealt with in a very individual way. What
> you tell the patient, how you tell the patient, when you tell the pat-
> ient, I think depends basically on the patient himself—on how you
> assess his need for information and what benefit this would be to
> him.

Certain considerations, or patient characteristics were considered by
the doctors to be of particular significance in the making of these judgements. For example, they believed that patients from the upper socio-
economic groups would not only want to know more but also, were
somehow thought to be better able to accept the truth and more likely
to display fortitude and retain their composure in the face of an alarming communication. Similar beliefs were held in relation to the patient's
perceived intelligence. More intelligent patients were attributed with a
greater desire to know the truth and because, as one doctor said, 'I
think more intelligent people tend to be better educated and know
that you can cure it', there was presumably less risk attached to telling
them. Other professed considerations included the patient's age, the
extent of his commitments, how aware the doctor perceived him to be,
and the doctor's assessment of his desire for information and probable
reaction to disclosure.

But, of course, as I have already indicated, decisions were not taken
in individual cases. It was just not possible to make such judgements
with any certainty of being correct. The intractable nature of the uncertainties endemic to such assessments precluded the implementation

of any policy geared to treating each case on its merits. The response to these uncertainties was not to disclose to any of the patients.

However, while asserting the individually based determinants of telling, the doctors themselves also simultaneously displayed an awareness, which was often relatively implicit, of their use of routine ways of communicating with patients. Firstly, they could articulate in abstract and general terms what their practices of telling were without reference to the non-clinical aspects of cases. Such general and abstract descriptions of what patients with particular types of condition were told would not have been possible had telling been individually based. In addition, though, they also acknowledged that what they termed 'set plans' or 'fixed patterns' governed their communication with patients:

> During your training as a doctor and handling malignant disease over the years you get a certain fixed pattern which is modified according to the psychological make-up of the patient.

> There is a plan which you generally adhere to. A particular patient with a particular disease is told a particular thing.

The doctors' awareness of the use of such routine devices would appear to be wholly inconsistent with their assertion that communication was based upon their assessment of individual patients. However, there was a sense in which what was communicated was influenced by their assessment of individuals. While the *substance* of what patients in the same category were told was constant the *detail* of what was communicated could differ. That is, although the meaning conveyed to patients in a particular category was equivalent in every case and no patient received a more explicit diagnosis or prognosis than others, the level of explanation and the terminology employed could vary in accordance with the doctor's perception of patients' ability to absorb information. This was the only sense in which communication could be said to be modified according to the doctor's assessment of particular individuals. But, even then, variations in what patients were told tended to be small and infrequent. In practice, what patients in the same category were told was remarkably similar in the great majority of cases.

However, although what the doctors communicated to patients depended only marginally upon their assessment of individuals, there is no doubt that such assessments were made. Inevitably the doctors would make judgements about patients in terms of how aware they were, whether they were anxious, how they would react to knowing, whether they would accept treatment and how much they wanted to know. Quite simply, they endeavoured to be prepared for possible reactions. This state of preparedness required the doctors to assess each patient on an individual basis. In doing so, they were engaged in a constant monitoring of patients' reactions and assessment of how they were likely to behave in future. My argument is simply that the substance of what was communicated to patients did not depend upon these conclusions. Communication was routinized and followed automatically from the allocation of cases to particular categories.

The Routinization of Communication

Routinization contributed to the management of communication in three main ways.

Firstly, it ensured consistency in the sort of information which a patient, or patients with similar conditions, received from any of the staff. This was particularly important in view of the fact that patients compared their conditions and progress with each other and occasionally attempted to trip up the medical staff by asking the same questions of different doctors.

Secondly, it absolved the doctors from having to take decisions in individual cases. The consultants maintained that what the patient was to be told was often decided in the weekly ward conferences. There, they said, a uniform story was constructed so that all the staff would tell the patient the same thing. However, no decision making on what to tell patients was observed either there or elsewhere. Nor, of course, was it necessary. Quite simply, the existence of the routines rendered such decision making redundant. The routines, and the typifications upon which they were based, dictated what patients were to be told. The staff had only to know the diagnosis and the treatment which the patient was to receive to be able to implement the appropriate routine. Furnished with the clinical details of the case and its proposed treatment, all staff members would follow the same routine prescriptions for telling. Everyone knew what to tell a patient with a particular condition, which was being treated in a particular way, at a particular stage of treatment. There was no decision to be taken. Given the uncertainty about patients' desire for information and possible reactions to being told, this effectively eliminated the possibility for error which would have existed had decisions been taken in individual cases. It ensured that patients who did not want to know or could not bear the news were never told. In addition, of course, the fact that responses to questions were also routinized meant that the doctors were also spared the potentially tricky business of having to think up answers on the spot.

The only decisions which were taken in ward conferences were decisions on treatment. There the patient's diagnosis, prognosis and course of treatment were discussed in detail. The weekly ward conferences were usually attended by the surgeons and radiotherapists, a radiologist whose main function was to interpret and comment upon X-rays, a haemotologist, the junior medical staff, the theatre sister, a sister or staff nurse from both male and female wards and, occasionally, a medical social worker. After the conference, all those attending went on a ward round together. The conference provided a forum in which members of the medical and nursing staff could congregate to learn about and discuss each case and where treatment could be decided upon in concert. They functioned both to inform the staff and to pool information for decision making on treatment. In this setting each individual's specialist knowledge could be brought to bear on the decision making process. Each case was reviewed in turn by one of the junior doctors with the consultants interjecting and raising problems, or points of interest, for discussion where appropriate. Discussion in these gatherings was concerned chiefly with questions of diagnosis and treatment. However, information on the patient's background, social and family circumstances, and 'state of mind' was relayed to the senior staff by the junior doctors and the nurses. The senior staff took the lead in decision making — the role of the other ranks being to provide information pertinent to the decisions which had to be taken. They did not make decisions. Although contributions from others may have influenced it, the ultimate decision rested with the consultant in charge of each case.

But not all treatment decisions were taken in the conferences. In fact only a minority were taken there. Decisions were often held in abeyance until after the conference and the ensuing ward round. Indeed, some decisions had to be delayed until the patient was seen by everyone. And, sometimes the doctors would change their minds after having seen the patient again. So discussion continued and decisions were made and revised both during and after the ward round. Clearly, it was difficult to take decisions at the bedside. Consequently they were usually taken elsewhere; for example, in the lift or corridor or over coffee. Nor, of course, could decision making be confined to one day of the week. Decisions had to be made as, and when, the need arose. So, the conference was where information was pooled and cases reviewed and discussed but not where all decisions were taken. Decision making might occur anywhere and at any time.

That decision making specifically about what patients should be told did not take place may have been implicitly recognized by the doctors. Consider the following extract:

> . . . what the patient is to be told depends also on what we intend doing to them. It's all linked with what your line of treatment is going to be. Now, the way this is resolved is that the line of treatment has got to be thrashed out first of all. And then, roughly what the patient is told, and this, I mean, in the majority of cases this is done in a sort of stereotyped way if you like . . . a particular patient with a particular disease is told a particular thing. If, however, in certain cases . . . this one case I remember in particular . . . there is disagreement over what the patient is told, the patient is told nothing, in fact, until it's threshed out by the members of staff exactly what she's going to be told. With this patient there was some degree of controversy as to whether she should have her leg amputated . . . she had a malignant melanoma of the leg and they were toying with the idea, or hadn't really decided until three or four days after she came in whether they would amputate or not. Clearly, if you haven't yet decided what you're going to do, how you're going to treat this, whether you're going to amputate the leg or not, you can't tell them what the condition is. It's only when the treatment, as far as you can see, has been threshed out, and the minor treatment to follow has been decided, that you can tell the patient. And, this is the important thing, the patient is told nothing until they're all in agreement as to what they should be told.

Throughout the above quotation we see that decisions about what to tell and decisions over treatment are regarded as part of the same process. The doctor is unable, nor does he consider it appropriate, to distinguish between the two. Decision making on what to tell the patient is discussed in terms of decisions about treatment. But of course, they did not constitute discrete processes and therefore could not be so distinguished. There was no decision making on telling *per se.* The appropriate form of communication followed automatically once the treatment had been decided upon. The doctor quoted above demonstrates an implicit awareness of this. It was precisely because they were so linked that decisions on treatment were perceived by the staff as also being decisions about what to tell. Hence the claim that decisions on telling were taken in ward conferences. But, only insofar as decisions were taken on treatment could decision making on telling be said to obtain. However, even collective decision making on treatment was not always necessary. As one doctor said, most conditions had a 'label' leading to a 'typical course of action'. So, usually, communication followed routinely from routine decisions about the method of treatment to be employed.

The third consequence of routinization was that it ensured that members of staff did not come into conflict over what patients should be told. The routines embodied certain rules concerning who could tell and what they could tell. Although any doctor could communicate with any patient in accordance with the appropriate routine, every consultant acknowledged that disclosure was the sole responsibility of the consultant in charge of the particular case. Likewise, the consultants' jurisdiction over telling was recognised and acceded to by the junior doctors. The rule that they should not tell was strictly adhered to. On no occasion did a junior doctor volunteer the diagnosis or prognosis to a patient. Junior doctors had, of course, to communicate with patients who were the responsibility of particular consultants. Routinization meant that they were able to do so without consulting their superiors about what to tell individual patients and in the knowledge that, because the routines contained only euphemistic reference to the patient's condition, what they said would not conflict with the consultant's policy. So, because the individual consultant's responsibility for telling his own patients was acknowledged by all, and because there was no decision making on telling, there was no scope for open conflict or disagreement either between different ranks in the medical hierarchy or between individual consultants.

Explicit instruction of junior doctors on what, or what not, to tell patients was regarded as unnecessary. They were expected to have learned how and what to communicate to patients during the course of their training and, thereafter, were meant to detect any differences in orientation in any particular ward through observation of the techniques employed by the consultants there. That they became conversant with how to communicate with patients without any formal instruction, either during training or upon attachment to a particular ward, was confirmed by the residents:

Well, nobody ever told me not to tell anybody or to tell anybody. I think you learn it through observing more than anything else. You just sniff it out—nobody ever said. You wouldn't start off by telling ... it would be an obvious way to antagonise people. And you learn this while you are a student anyway, I think. That what is told to the patient, if it's serious, is done by the senior member of staff, and you're not supposed to say anything else really.

The consultants' jurisdiction over telling was absolute in the hospital context. No one had any right to interefere with what they chose to tell their patients nor did anyone do so. Similarly, though, outside agencies did not exert any influence upon their practices either. In particular, general practitioners' views on telling were not taken into account. Because the consultants believed that the GPs' orientations, in the main, did not differ to any marked degree from their own, and because they did not really know the detailed policies of individual GPs anyway, the question of tailoring what the patient was told to whatever preference his GP might have had did not arise. However, had they been aware that a GP had a policy which conflicted with their own, it would almost certainly not have influenced what they told his patients. While in hospital, the patient was regarded as the sole responsibility of the consultant, his authority being total in all matters relating to his care.

> The GP is in charge in the community and the consultant in the hospital. The GP may inform the consultant of specific factors about the patient and advise on some matters and the consultant may inform the GP of what he has told the patient. But, in the hospital, the consultant tells the patient what he feels it is best for him to know.

But, of course, if a GP had had a policy of telling, this would not have been jeopardised by the policy of not disclosing in the hospital. If the ward policy had been one of telling, the position might have been very different. In that case, the GP's views might have been an important consideration. The consultants might not have wanted to offend or alienate them by informing their patients. The GP could always tell his patients if he wanted to, but he could not 'untell' them. So, in a sense, the policy of the consultants on Ward 4C ultimately left the decision on telling to the GP. In the few cases where patients were told, given that the consultants would only tell when they had no alternative, there was no scope for accommodating GPs' preferences when that point was reached. If the consultant had to tell, he had to tell.

From the argument presented in this chapter it is clear that uncertainty played a major part in structuring the form and content of communication with patients in the present context. While the doctors believed that some patients should be told they could not establish, with any certainty, whether individuals genuinely wanted to know or how they would react. And, given the anticipated consequences of informing inappropriate persons, they had to be sure before doing so. The adoption of routine procedures, the central concern of which was the avoidance of disclosure to all patients, provided a way of coping with these uncertainties consistent with their belief that the great majority of patients did not want to know and would not benefit from disclosure. The next two chapters examine the routine ways in which the medical staff managed communication with patients.

Notes

1. This observation is based upon reports which the author received from doctors, medical students and nurses who had attended other wards in the hospital.
2. This belief would appear to be widely held (Oken 1961, p. 1123).
3. Note the similarity between this principle and one portrayed by Scheff. He found that, in the event of diagnostic uncertainty, the majority of doctors operate with the principle that to judge a sick person well is more to be avoided than to judge a well person sick. Scheff, T. J. 'Decision Rules, Types of Error, and Their Consequences in Medical Diagnosis'; *Behavioural Science 8*, pp. 97-107, 1963.
4. Apart from the doctors' natural reluctance to practise outright deceit, there were important practical reasons for the avoidance of lying. If the doctors had told patients lies, or if they had lied to some patients, they would have had to remember, or record, what each individual patient had been told for fear of contradicting themselves in subsequent encounters. Moreover, lying would have created problems if, and when, more frank discussion became necessary or if the patient became aware of the truth in some other way. Whereas a half-truth would enable the doctor to expand upon it and provided a basis for truthful discussion at a future date, an outright lie would not. If frankness was subsequently called for, a lie would have to be retracted. This would constitute an admission of deceit, reveal the doctor in a poor light, and probably destroy the patient's confidence and trust in him.
5. This finding is consistent with other work on the management of uncertainty. (Scheff 1963; Roth 1958).
6. For discussion of typifications see T.J. Scheff (1968) and D. Sudnow (1968).

3 ROUTINE PROCEDURES FOR TELLING

There were two distinct sets of routines employed by the doctors in their communication with patients. One set related to information *volunteered* to patients while the other was concerned with *responses* to questioning by them. In this chapter I examine those routines associated with what was volunteered to patients. As I have already indicated, the routines were grounded in typifications of different types of condition. Conditions were allocated to particular stereotypical categories on the basis of their degree of severity. Each category of conditions had attached to it a particular routine way of communicating with patients at particular stages of their treatment. In operating these routines different doctors might inform the same patient in slightly different ways while the same doctor might inform patients with the same or similar conditions in a different manner. However, while the detail of communications might vary, in substance what patients in the same category were told was equivalent since the meaning conveyed to all was the same. With every sort of case the doctor attempted to minimise, as far as possible, the implied seriousness of the condition although, as we will see, certain contingencies of the case, primarily its severity, constrained the extent to which he could do so.

The routines associated with what was volunteered to patients were differentially appropriate to the following main categories of conditions: (1) simple conditions, including both non-malignant growths and easily cured cancers; (2) conditions which the doctor believed to be probably benign; (3) more serious cancers of uncertain or unfavourable prognosis; and, (4) very serious conditions requiring major operative procedures. Each of these will be examined in turn.

Simple Conditions
Communication with patients with simple conditions was relatively straightforward and unproblematic. Simple cancers and benign conditions could be incorporated within the same category because, to the doctors, they were equally innocuous. A simple malignancy presented them with no greater problem, in terms of cure, than did the removal of a non-malignant condition. Moreover, with both types of condition their main objective was the same: to emphasise their non-serious nature to patients and to assure them that they would not recur. Thus, one

routine sufficed for both.

When he first saw the patient, the doctor would attempt to assure him that his condition was not dangerous. However, in doing so, he faced a problem of achieving a balance between suggesting the removal of the growth and discounting its seriousness. There was a danger that the fact that the doctor had decided to treat the condition might in itself suggest to the patient that it must therefore be serious, particularly if he suspected that he might have cancer. This was resolved by justifying treatment on cosmetic grounds, because the growth was a nuisance or as a prophylactic measure.[1]

> I don't think this is a serious sort of mole, but because you're liable to injure it shaving, we'll take it away for you.

> Now this isn't anything to worry about. It's not dangerous. But because it's unsightly we'll remove it for you.

> Well Mr Forbes, I think we should get rid of this ulcer for you. It's nothing to worry about at the moment but if it was left it could give you a bit of trouble in the future. So I think it's best to remove it for you. But, as I say, it's not serious at the moment. Look at it as a safeguard.

In this way, the doctor disclaimed the importance of the growth other than as an inconvenience or because it could potentially give trouble if it were left. Following its removal the patient was again assured that it was not serious and should not cause any further trouble. 'Now, as I said before your operation, that thing was nothing to worry about. It won't trouble you again.' 'That thing on your cheek was perfectly harmless. It won't come back again.'

So, from the outset, patients with simple, easily cured cancers, or conditions which were clearly non-malignant, could be informed categorically that they were unproblematic. However, conditions which the doctor, in his clinical judgement, considered to be only *probably* benign were a different matter and required a different approach.

Probably Benign

Unlike the previous category, here there was a possibility that the condition could be serious. The patient had to be prepared for this. The procedure employed had therefore to be slightly different from that outlined above. Initially, the doctor could not state definitely that the condition was not serious. Prior to establishment of the precise nature of the condition the problem which he faced lay in striking the correct balance between conveying to the patient that the growth was probably harmless while at the same time leaving open the possibility that it might not be without alarming him unduly. This he achieved by always including in his communication with such patients some reference to the fact that the condition might not be harmless while at the same time emphasising that this was thought to be a rather unlikely possibility.

> Now we think this is a harmless thing but there is a slight chance that it might not be. So we'll take you to theatre and have a look at it under a microscope and if it looks at all suspicious we will have to remove the breast. But, as I said, we think it's harmless, and I don't think that will be necessary. So I wouldn't worry about it.

In order to reassure the patient, the doctor would often express the chances of the condition being innocuous in percentage terms. 'I think we should have you in and snip that thing out. The chances are 99% that it's just a little cyst but we can never be 100% sure.' After the operation, when the condition had been confirmed as benign, the patient was left in no doubt that it was harmless. 'This thing that we removed was quite simple. We had it examined under the microscope and there was nothing dangerous about it. There was no abnormality there. It was quite a simple thing and it won't bother you again.'

Occasionally, the doctor would use the term 'malignant' to emphasise to the patient that the condition was benign.

> Dr Shoemark[2]: We had a look at your X-rays and found a little thing blocking one of the ducts. It's what we've been looking for for some time.
> Patient: So you'll take it out?
> Dr Shoemark: Yes. But it's nothing to worry about. It's not malignant or anything like that.
> Patient: Oh, that's what's been on my mind since I came in.
> Dr Shoemark: It's more like a little wart. We'll just cut it out. We won't remove the breast.
> Patient: (smiling) I should hope not.

Malignancies of Uncertain or Unfavourable Prognosis

A different routine was observed by the doctors when communicating

with patients with all cancers other than the simple ones or those requiring major surgical intervention. Those malignancies were all serious to
some degree and of uncertain or unfavourable prognosis. They constituted the bulk of the doctors' work. What the doctor had to achieve
here was to convey to the patient that his condition was serious enough
to necessitate an operation or prolonged course of treatment while, at
the same time, leaving him with hope and not alarming him.

The doctor required the patient's consent at two crucial stages: he
had to get the patient to agree to come into hospital in the first place,
and once there, had to acquire his consent for an operation or treatment. Therefore, he had to convince him, firstly, that hospitalization
was necessary and, secondly, that treatment of the condition was essential. But, in doing so, he had to strike a balance between impressing the
seriousness of the condition on the patient, sufficient to get his consent
at different stages, and not alarming him. Clearly, he did not want to
tell the patient that he thought he might have cancer. When persuading
patients to come into hospital, he was often able to avoid doing so by
professing to be uncertain about the diagnosis but adding that it probably had to be treated, whatever it was.

We'll have to get you into hospital to find out about this. We'll have
to get something done about it. I'm not sure yet what, but it is
certainly something which must be treated.

Well, you've got an ulcer there and you'll have to come into hospital
for treatment. We will also have to do some X-rays and tests to
determine its true nature. But it's the sort of thing that has to be
taken seriously.

In this way the doctor could indicate that the condition had to be
treated, and thus get the patient to come into hospital, without having
to reveal that he suspected that it could be malignant.

Professions, or implications, of uncertainty were also used to avoid
the rendering of an explicit diagnosis when obtaining patients' consent
for an operation or treatment. Sometimes the diagnosis had not been
ascertained prior to the requirement of consent and the doctor could
genuinely claim to be uncertain of it. Often the patient's diagnosis was
not established until he was in theatre ready to undergo an operation,
the biopsy, and the form of surgical intervention which its result
implied, being carried out during the same operating session. In such
cases, the doctor could indicate quite openly that he was uncertain of

the nature of the condition and therefore, by implication, was unable to tell the patient what he had. But, in order to obtain the patient's consent for what could be a quite extensive operation, the doctor had to concede that his condition might be serious. At the same time, of course, he did not wish to reveal the possible diagnosis or cause him undue alarm. He was able to avoid doing either, and to acquire the patient's consent, by referring to what might be found in an euphemistic way and by informing him that, even if his condition was only *potentially* serious, they would proceed with surgery.

> You've got a bit of thickening there. We'll take a bit of it out and have a look at it under the microscope and, if there are any suspicious cells there, we'll have to do a more radical procedure. Even if there's a small chance that there might be, we'll have to remove your breast just to be sure.

> When we take you to theatre, we'll take a bit of this out and have a look at it under the microscope and, if any cells look even as if they might become nasty, we will remove the breast. We always try to err on the side of safety.

Usually, though, the diagnosis was known in advance of the decision on treatment. This was certainly so where an operation was not the selected form of treatment or where a biopsy had been taken prior to the decision to operate. In these circumstances, the rendering of a diagnosis could not be postponed by openly professing to be uncertain of it. The doctor could not legitimately claim to be unsure nor would the patient accept that he was proceeding without knowing what he was treating. Nevertheless, while it was not professed outright, uncertainty was still employed as a device for avoiding the use of an explicit diagnosis. Its use was simply more covert and subtle than an open confession by the doctor that he did not know. Communication was conducted by means of euphemisms which ascribed a certain ambiguity to the diagnosis. Some measure of uncertainty was implicit in the use of terms like 'suspicious cells' or 'activity' which implied that the diagnosis was somewhat equivocal.[3] In this way, the euphemisms not only provided the doctors with a way of communicating with patients without having to refer explicitly to their diagnosis, they also, with their implied uncertainty, provided a justification for not giving one. In addition, it was felt that such euphemistic accounts of the nature of his condition would also leave the suspicious patient with the hope, or impression, that the diagnosis was equivocal and that he might not have cancer after all. The other element of the doctors' technique was to portray the patient's condition as being only potentially serious, the implication being that they had caught it in time. That the treatment would be successful was taken for granted. Patients were informed of the decision to operate in the following way:

> We've got the report back on that and it's certainly active. So you've got to have it dealt with, otherwise it's going to cause you trouble, either in a year or two, maybe sooner if it became a bit more active. So we'll remove it for you sometime next week.

> Well, Mrs Finnie, our tests show that there are some suspicious cells in that thing so we think it best if we remove it, and some of the area round about, because it could become dangerous if it was left.

The decision to treat the patient by means of non-surgical forms of intervention was imparted in a similar way.

> Well Mr Ogilvie, the X-rays showed that you have some inflamation on your lung. Now, this has to be treated or it could turn nasty. So we've decided to give you some radiotherapy to get rid of it for you.

Sometimes the patient received a combination of treatments:

> Now, as you know, we found some activity in that lump. We have decided to give you a course of injections followed by X-ray treatment to get rid of it for you. We find this combination of treatment is very effective indeed. The drug will soften the inflamation and the X-rays will take over from that.

However, certain forms of treatment were more difficult to explain. With hormone ablative procedures (adrenalectomy, oopherectomy, pituitary ablation) the doctors had the additional problem of explaining to the patient why they should be operating upon a part of his anatomy other than where the condition was manifest. They had somehow to connect the operation with the condition in their explanation. There was another problem. These procedures were undertaken for more serious disorders, usually where secondary deposits of the disease were involved. Moreover, the patient probably had some awareness of the relatively serious nature of his illness: his symptoms were often considerably more striking and troublesome than those associated with many of the primary lesions and he was often on a second or subsequent admission for treatment of his condition. He probably knew that something was badly wrong and that something had to be done about it. His condition could not, therefore, be presented as being only potentially serious. Nevertheless, the principles underlying communication with those patients were the same as for the others in this category: the condition was described by means of euphemisms; its immediate severity was played down; and the prospect of cure was treated as being relatively unproblematic.

> We've decided that to cure your trouble we'll remove your ovaries and the glands at the top of your kidneys. They give out hormones which we think are responsible for your condition. They're no use to you—you won't miss them—and when we do this it should get rid of the pain you're having.

> Well Mrs Field, we've got the results of our tests and it seems that you have some suspicious cells which are causing the trouble. We've had a discussion about it and we have decided to take away the gland at the top of your nose. These cells depend for their growth upon a particular hormone which is secreted by this gland and we hope to stop the cells dividing so rapidly and to slow up their activity by taking the gland away.

Once they had had their operation, or had completed their treatment, the doctors sought to give the patients an assessment of their condition in such a way that they would not worry after discharge. However, they had to do so without explicitly saying that they were cured unless, of course, they were certain of this. In most cases the doctors could not be absolutely certain and such a positive prognosis could have rebounded on them. Instead, patients were informed *by implication* that their prognosis was good. After their operation patients were not told that their condition had been malignant. Again, only euphemistic reference was made to their illness. The operation was justified in terms of the potential seriousness of the condition and of erring on the side of caution.

> Well Miss Barraclough, that mass in your breast contained some suspicious cells so we thought it was best to remove it. It's just as well that you had it done because in a year or so it would probably have

been serious. We also took away some glands from your armpit. Al-
thought there didn't seem to be anything in them, it's always best
to be on the safe side.

That was certainly active and would have been dangerous if we had
left it there. There's none of it left though. That's why we did such
a wide excision.

By indicating that the condition was only potentially serious or by
implying that it had been caught in time the doctors could convey to
patients the impression that the prognosis was good without explicitly
saying that they were cured.

However, in some cases it was necessary to treat the patient's condition with radiotherapy in addition to, and after, surgery or even to
perform a second operation. The doctor had to try to ensure that the
fact that these additional procedures were being carried out did not suggest to the patient that his condition had turned out to be more serious
than had been thought initially. They were therefore presented as being
ways of making certain.

There was a bit of activity about this so we have removed the
breast and the glands in your armpit. We will get the final report on
the glands in a week and, if they are a bit inflamed or involved at all,
then we will add on some X-ray treatment as well just to make
doubly sure that everything is going to be all right. Don't worry
about it though. It's just to make absolutely certain.

We're going to give you some X-ray treatment as a precaution—just
in case there are some cells that shouldn't be there. We think it's unlikely, but we do it just to be on the safe side.

There was some activity about this when we removed it. There's a
one in a hundred chance that anything could be left but, just to make
sure, we'll do another operation and remove the area around it. We
always like to be on the safe side.

Patients who had been treated by means of radiotherapy or drugs
were often discharged before there was any marked sign of improvement in their health or, at least, before the disease could be said to
have been eradicated. Again, though, they were led to believe that a
favourable outcome was expected. During the course of their treatment,

such patients received encouraging information on their progress—'the X-ray showed a great improvement', 'the results of the tests were good', 'that's much better'—the intention being to make the patient feel that the treatment was working, as it usually did to varying degrees. Upon discharge, the patients were not only informed that their health would continue to improve after the treatment had stopped and they had gone home, it was also implied in an almost taken for granted way, that it would eventually culminate in a cure. After all, that was ostensibly the ultimate aim of the treatment, it was working, and therefore the question of cure need not arise. 'Now, the treatment keeps on working after you have stopped getting it, and you'll continue to get better after you've gone home.' In this way, the doctors sought to discharge patients who believed that they were well on the way to being cured, without having to render an explicit prognosis.

Finally, all patients who had been treated for cancer were asked to report at an outpatient clinic, at intervals after their discharge, so that the doctors could keep them under surveillance in case there was a recurrence of the disease. This posed the potential problem of how to explain to the patient why he should be required to attend a follow-up clinic when he was supposed to be cured. This was resolved by justifying such periodic checks in terms of 'making sure' and by, at the same time, emphasising that any further problems were thought to be extremely unlikely.

We would like to see you at the clinic every so often just in case you have any trouble. As I said, we don't expect you to have any trouble, we expect you to get better, but just in case.

Now, we'll see you at the clinic every so often just to keep an eye on it. We don't think that it will give you any more bother. We're pretty sure it will be all right but it's just as well to keep a check on it.

Conditions Requiring Major Surgery

The final routine was employed in communicating with patients who required a major operation such as an amputation. This routine was characterized by a gradual build-up to the announcement that a major operation was required and an accompanying indication of the severity of the condition which was in excess of that rendered to patients who did not have to undergo such a radical procedure. The doctor had to get the patient to agree to submit to surgery of a major kind so he had to present him with a very good reason for doing so. Consequently, the severity of the condition had to be indicated to a greater extent than with other cancers.

When he was seen as an outpatient the patient was told that he would have to come into hospital to be examined but that his condition would 'certainly require treatment' or was 'something which had to be taken seriously'. Once the patient was in hospital and once the doctors were aware of the probable action they would have to take, the gradual build-up began in earnest. The reasons for bringing the patient to a gradual awareness that his condition was serious were twofold. Firstly, to shield him from the shock of a sudden disclosure: 'we have decided to amputate your leg'. Secondly, to organise the patient's acceptance of the operation. A patient who was aware that his condition was serious would more readily accept a drastic remedy. As part of the process of preparation the doctors would let the patient know that they were anxious about his condition. A series of X-rays and tests would be carried out and the proferring of the results of these, to the patient, would be used to stress the serious nature of the condition.

> We got the results of the test and that thing is certainly active. Now we're still waiting for the results of the other tests, but if they show that it's malignant, or going malignant, we will have to do an extensive operation. It may even involve having to remove your leg.

So, the patient was, at that stage, warned that major surgical intervention might be required. Ultimately the doctor had to break the news that a major operation was definitely necessary. But, in doing so he did not tell the patient that he had cancer. Instead, he would inform him that his condition was 'going malignant' or would 'turn cancerous'. So again the condition was characterised as being potentially serious the difference this time being that the nature of the projected development was stated explicitly. Such an assessment, while not as threatening as a definite diagnosis of cancer, was sufficiently so to enable the doctor to acquire the patient's consent for the operation.

> Well, this is really nasty and we've got to do something or it could be a danger to your life if it were left. That thing is definitely going malignant so we've decided that the only realistic course of action is to remove your leg in case it spreads.

> Now Mr Fry, you know we were worried about this. Well, we've got

the results of the tests and there are some cells in your leg which, if
your leg is not taken off, will turn cancerous. So we've decided that
the only way to make sure that you don't have any more trouble
is to remove your leg.

After the operation the patient was assured that it went well and
should be successful.

These, then, were the routine procedures associated with what was
volunteered to patients. They were differentially appropriate to different
categories of conditions. However, the category to which the patient's
condition belonged did not always remain constant during his stay in
hospital. For example, a patient might be admitted with a suspected
benign condition, and prepared accordingly, only to have it turn out to
be malignant. Or, conversely, a suspected malignancy might turn out
to be benign. In the event of changes in diagnosis or prognosis, the
doctors simply switched to the routine appropriate to the revised category of condition.

Having outlined the role played by routinization in managing the
information volunteered to patients, certain other aspects of the control of information and the management of patients' awareness are
examined below.

Timing

The timing of communication, or when patients were told certain things,
was considered by the doctors to be important. Information was imparted to patients gradually and in stages. They were not told everything
at once because it was believed that it would be too much for them to
take, and too much for them to comprehend and remember. So, on
admission, patients were not informed of the possible outcomes of the
proposed investigations or of the alternative forms of treatment which
they might have to undergo. At first the patient was simply told that
tests had to be carried out and only later would he be given the results
of these and the decision on the method of treatment to be employed.
Similarly, when they were informed of the decision to operate, patients
were not simultaneously told that there was a possibility of additional
treatment to follow.

Now, we don't say to patients, 'We are going to do this and you
might have X-ray therapy afterwards.' It would be an awful blow to
a patient to say, 'Right, we are going to do this. If it is nasty we will
remove the breast and after a day or two we will get a report on the

glands. If they are involved, you will have to get X-ray treatment too.' That is an awful lot for them to accept at one time. Yet we get them to accept all this by timing it. And, of course, if you say, 'We are going to operate on that', anything else you say at that time is often superfluous. It just doesn't sink in.

So, patients were not, for example, informed that they were likely to get radiotherapy until after their operation. Nor were they told this immediately after surgery, although they were prepared for the possibility of it at that time. This gave patients time to recover before being informed that they were definitely to receive additional treatment and, it was hoped, also helped to soften the blow.

When we have operated on them, and we know that the glands are involved clinically and that the patient has got to have X-ray treatment, we don't say to the patient immediately after the operation, 'You have got to have a course of X-ray treatment lasting three weeks to a month.' What we say to them is, 'Now, there was a bit of activity about this, we have removed the breast and we will get the final report on the glands in a week. If they are at all infected, we will add on some X-ray treatment just to make sure.'

Timing was also regarded as being important in informing patients of the results of their operations. The patient was not normally told about the operation until the following day. It was felt that, if they were told immediately after the operation while still in a groggy state, they would probably forget it. The exception to this was if the patient had a benign condition. They would often be informed of this while barely conscious. The good news would be repeated the following morning to ensure comprehension.

. . . when you tell them the result of the operation is very important. If you tell them immediately post-operatively, they forget it. If the lump was malignant, you leave it till the next day to tell them. There's not much point in giving them bad news too early. If it's benign, you tell them as quickly as possible. This is, in many ways, because one likes telling good news instead of bad.

Just as the content of communication was routinely determined, so were the stages at which information was imparted to patients. A set pattern governed the times at which patients were given certain types of information. The purpose behind the timing of information, or giving it in stages, was to minimise the impact which the simultaneous delivery of a number of potentially threatening pieces of information might have had on the patient.

Diversionary Tactics

Certain tactics for forestalling questioning by patients and for managing cues were, of course, built into the routines which governed what was to be volunteered to them. For example, we have already seen that a constant concern of the doctors was to give the patients hope and that this was reflected in all their communication with them. By feeding the patient with optimistic pieces of information both prior and subsequent to his treatment, the doctors may have hoped effectively to pre-empt any questions which he otherwise might have asked. Similarly, simply by not giving the explicit diagnosis, they may have forestalled possible enquiries about the prognosis. Had the patient been informed that he had cancer, questions relating to the outlook might have assumed greater significance for him. The doctors had some awareness of the utility of this technique.

> But usually I would try to forestall them by telling them before they asked. If you go along to them as soon as possible and say that the tests showed some nasty cells so we had to take the breast away, or something like that, you see, then you cut them short before they have the chance to start worrying or before they'd ask.

In addition, though, certain diversionary tactics were employed to assist in the control of patients' awareness. One such approach was to concentrate upon the patient's symptoms or upon epiphenomonal disorders associated with his main condition, (for example, the collection of fluid in the pleural cavity with lung cancer), in an effort to divert his attention from his underlying problem.

> You've got some fluid there and that's what's causing the breathlessness. But we'll take it away this afternoon and you'll feel much better.

> We're going to put you on a course of drugs to stop the fluid accumulating in your lung. Once we've seen the chest films, we'll see if there's any more fluid to come off. Once we've done that, we'll start you on the pills. The fluid that's accumulating there is the cause of all

your symptoms and, if we stop it accumulating, you'll feel much better.

In the above examples, the doctor was not telling any lies. The collection of fluid was indeed responsible for the patients' symptoms and, upon its removal, they would undoubtedly feel better. He simply omitted to mention the underlying cause, that is, what caused the fluid to collect in the first place. The accumulation of fluid was thus treated as if it were an independent condition. In the second quotation, although drugs might serve to prevent the collection of fluid, they would do so by acting against its underlying cause: the malignancy.

Full use was also made of any non-malignant complaint which a patient might have in addition to his malignancy. It was observed that, in interaction with such patients, the doctors would often concentrate upon their non-malignant condition to the relative exclusion of the other. In this way, they could not only partially divert the patient's attention from his main illness but could also, by implication, play down the importance of the more serious condition. If the doctors appeared to pay as much, or more, attention to an evidently relatively innocuous complaint, then why should the patient be too worried about his main condition? However, they had to be careful that, in stressing the other condition, they did not raise patient fears that *it* was serious. So, it was not portrayed as being important in itself. It was simply stressed relative to the malignant condition. The innocuous nature of the non-malignant complaint was continually emphasized.

Humour

In order to display confidence in their ability to treat the condition and to instil optimism in the patient by playing down the seriousness of the illness, another device frequently employed by the doctors was humour. Through the use of humour they hoped to make the patient feel that, if they were able to joke, their condition could not be too serious and the doctors could not have any doubts about being able to treat it successfully. These jokes were usually related to topics other than the patient's condition, the latter not being regarded as an appropriate subject for humourous comment unless it was a very simple one. 'My goodness, that's a funny thing on your ear. You could almost hang your hat on it.' Occasionally, one of the surgeons would conduct what he termed 'a social type of ward round' where he would attempt, by means of humour, to raise ward morale. On such rounds he might have a joke for every single patient on the ward—quite a comic feat. All this is not to say that joking was a perpetual feature of communication with patients. It was not. Indeed, some patients were regarded as being too ill to joke with. Humour was used intermittently and where appropriate. At the same time, though, the doctors were careful not to belittle the patient's condition or to appear to be treating it lightly. Such an ap- proach could have undermined the patient's confidence in them. So, while they attempted to create an atmosphere of confidence and optim- ism through an attitude of relative lightheartedness, this was never allowed to transcend their basic approach to the patient's condition which remained manifestly conscientious and respectful.

> We wisecrack a lot with them. We discuss what they're doing and joke with them. I think this is part of their treatment. I suppose the impression the patient would get would be, 'Well, they don't seem to be worried about my condition. They seem to be quite confident.' But we don't belittle what they have got. We treat them and their symptoms and their condition with a certain amount of respect and firmness but also with a good degree of sympathy, but not going beyond a certain level in either respect. We try to instil into them some confidence that everything is going to be dealt with adequately. But, at the same time, we let them know that we are not treating their condition lightly.

Humour was also used by the doctors when discussing patients' con- ditions among themselves. It served as a tension release mechanism. 'If we didn't laugh at it, we would go mad. But we laugh at the lump, not at the patient.'

As we have seen, the routine forms of communication, and their con- comitants, associated with what was volunteered to patients, embodied certain attempts to forestall questioning, in particular by presenting the patient's condition in as optimistic a way as possible. However, despite this, patients did ask questions and make demands upon the doctors to reveal more about their condition than they were willing to volunteer. The routine ways of handling questions and pressures from patients are the subject of the next chapter.

Notes

1. In the case of the non-malignant conditions, the unsightly or inconvenient nat- ure of the growth was often the doctor's real reason for removing it.

2. The Doctors' names are all fictitious and applied randomly in order to minimise the possibility of identifying individual respondents.
3. This particular manifestation of the use of uncertainty is examined in greater detail in Chapter 4.

4 ROUTINE RESPONSES

Just as what was volunteered to patients was routinized, so was the information which they received in response to enquiries. For the doctors the same concerns as governed what they voluntarily told patients underlay their responses to questioning. They did not want to alarm them or destroy their hope. This, of course, implied avoidance of direct disclosure except in those cases where the patient could be said genuinely to want to know and to be capable of taking the news. However, as I argued earlier, there was no way in which the doctors could be certain of this. Even the fact that a patient asked did not constitute proof that he wanted to know, still less that he would receive disclosure with reasonable equanimity. He might simply be seeking reassurance. There was no way of distinguishing such a request from a demand for the truth. Moreover, while the question, 'Do I have cancer?' was quite explicit and while certain others, for example, 'Has it spread?' or 'Will it come back?' might be said to display an awareness of certain features of malignancy, those which were posed most frequently, such as, 'What is it?' or 'What's wrong?', were the sorts of questions which any patient might ask in innocence of the reply which he might receive.

Given that they could not be certain that the patient 'really' wanted to know the truth or could stand to be told, even if he asked outright, the employment of routine responses geared to avoiding disclosure in *all* cases provided a way of coping with this. While it might have been hard on those patients who genuinely wanted to know, this did ensure that patients who did not want to know were never informed. The routine responses were consistent with what was routinely volunteered to patients and, indeed, often the content of what was volunteered to them and what they were told in response to questioning was very similar. The routines were based upon typifications of questions and conditions. A particular type of question posed by a patient with a particular type of condition elicited a particular type of response. Replies were framed in such a way as to obviate further questioning by the patient. I begin by examining the routine responses to questions relating to the diagnosis.

The Diagnosis

The response to questions about the diagnosis depended in part upon when they were asked. If a patient asked what he had before clinical certainty had been established, the doctor's reply was relatively unproblematic. He did not know the diagnosis for certain and therefore could not give one. The patient was told that he did not know and that tests would have to be done to find out. The doctor could not, however, plead ignorance once investigations had been carried out. At that stage, in response to questions like, 'What is it?' or 'What did you find?', he sought refuge in an euphemistic response. Again he would usually present the condition as being only potentially harmful and, in doing so, negate for the patient the importance of obtaining a more precise definition of it.

> Well, there is an ulcer there as you can see. Our tests showed that there is a bit of activity about it. So we have decided to remove it in case it becomes dangerous in time.

> Well, as you know there was a lump there. The test we did showed some nasty cells in it so we thought it was best to remove the breast. It should be all right now though.

> Well, it's a little growth and we've decided to remove it in case it becomes troublesome.

Although most patients did not enquire further, the responses to these questions were sometimes challenged. When they were challenged, the doctor had to be more explicit in his reply. This usually involved telling a patient that 'it was going malignant' or 'would have turned into a cancer', again implying that the condition was not immediately serious. Very seldom did patients pursue the matter any further than that.

> Patient: What do you mean when you say there are some nasty cells there?
> Dr Chisholm: Well, it means that it might have turned into a cancer if it had been left. That's why we removed it.

> Patient: What exactly do you mean by 'suspicious cells'?
> Mr Moorhead: Well, they were going malignant and it would have been dangerous to have left it. That's why we operated—to make sure that you wouldn't have any more trouble.

Questions relating to treatment or investigations might also have been designed to elicit information about the diagnosis. One set of questions related to why certain tests were carried out. They were explained in terms of being 'routine' or 'to find out what it is'. The possible diagnosis was not mentioned.

Patient: What was that for doctor?
Dr Barron: Well, that was a thermogram. It's a new technique we're perfecting to see if it can show up a nasty spot.

Patient: Why did I get all these X-rays?
.Dr Dunlop: Oh, it's just a routine that we do to all patients. It's also a good screening device. And, of course, as you're getting an anaesthetic, we like to make sure your chest's OK.

Questions about the purpose of treatment also received an euphemistic response, 'It's to reduce that swelling' or, 'It's for the inflamation you've got here. It's to get rid of that.'

Although it was comparatively rare, patients did sometimes ask the more pointed questions, 'Is it cancer?' and 'Is it malignant?' They were given neither a positive nor a negative answer. There were a number of ways in which this could be achieved consistent with the same type of routine response. Again the condition was referred to in terms of euphemisms or its potential seriousness.

Well, it's an active sort of growth and it could be troublesome if we didn't treat it in the correct way. It could turn very nasty in a year or two if it was left. That's why we decided to remove it for you.

Well, it could certainly have become malignant if it had been left. That's why we took it away. It shouldn't trouble you now though.

Well, if it was left it would certainly grow into a big ulcer which would continue to grow. But we'll easily get rid of it for you and you needn't worry about it. But it is active, there's no doubt about that, and it would be stupid to leave it.

Most of the time, then, questions relating to the diagnosis were relatively easily handled by the doctors through the use of routine responses which were characterized by avoidance of explicit disclosure and implied that the condition was potentially serious and that treatment was of a prophylactic nature. These responses usually succeeded in preventing further questioning by patients by playing down the present severity of their condition and giving them the impression that their illness was not as threatening as they might have imagined.

Although questions about the diagnosis might carry an implicit request for information about the prognosis, other questions related more explicitly to it.

The Prognosis

During the course of the study no patient asked if they were going to die or how long they had to live. However, they did ask other questions relating to their prognosis. Questions such as, 'Will I be all right now?', 'Did you get it all?', 'Will it come back?' and 'Has it spread?' were designed to find out how bad their condition was, and hence what the outlook was likely to be, short of ascertaining whether it would prove fatal. When faced with those questions, the doctors' objectives were to ensure, through their replies, that the patient would retain hope and not worry unduly. This was achieved by responding to patients in such a way as to indicate a hopeful outlook. Indeed, the prognosis *might* be good. The doctors could not be absolutely certain that it was not. This provided the justification for emphasizing the hopeful aspects of the outlook. The doctors sought to give as optimistic a reply as possible. The extent to which they could do so depended upon their perception of the prognosis. The more certain they were that the prognosis was likely to be good, the more certain and optimistic were their replies. Where the doctor was confident of a favourable prognosis he would un-equivocally tell the patient so.

> Patient: Did you get it all?
> Dr Shoemark: Oh yes, we're quite sure, quite sure.

> Patient: Is it all clear now?
> Dr Ogston: Yes.
> Patient: Positive?
> Dr Ogston: Oh yes. That's why we took so much away—to make sure we got it all. That's why we had to take the whole breast off.

When he was less certain of the prognosis, or where he believed the outlook to be bad, while the doctor still wanted to present a hopeful picture, he had also to guard against telling a deliberate untruth which could rebound on him at a later date. He had to strike a balance between giving the patient to believe that the outlook was good and not telling him an outright lie. This was usually achieved by injecting some measure of uncertainty into his response.

Patient: But it'll just come back somewhere else?
Dr Barron: Oh no. Not necessarily. We think we got it all. I don't
    think there's anything for you to worry about.

Patient: Did you get all of it out?
Dr Samuel: Oh yes, I think so.
Patient: There aren't any roots left?
Dr Samuel: Oh no, we're pretty certain there aren't. It shouldn't
    trouble you again.

Enquiries about the purpose of supplementary treatment might also incorporate some reference to the outlook. The response to these questions again contained a trace of uncertainty, the doctors trying to create the impression that the prognosis was good without stating definitely that the patient was cured. The patient was informed that the additional treatment was simply a precautionary measure and should not be taken to indicate that their condition was bad or that the disease had not been eradicated.

Patient: Does this mean that you haven't got it all?
Mr Donald: Well, we're almost certain we've got everything. We're
    just giving you this course of treatment to wipe out any cells that
    might have got left. You should be all right then. It's just to make
    sure.

Patient: Why do I have to get radiotherapy? Does this mean I'm not
    all clear?
Dr Craib: Oh, no. It's just a precaution. We're just doing it as a safe-
    guard, just in case some cells have been left. This will make sure
    that we get them all.

While the routine responses to questions about both the diagnosis and prognosis usually succeeded in their objective of discouraging or obviating further enquiry, such accounts of the patient's condition were sometimes successfully challenged and superseded by disclosure.

Challenging the Routines

As we have seen, the routine ways of managing patients' enquiries were such that any questions about the diagnosis or prognosis could be accommodated by an euphemistic set of responses. While this provided the ideal coping mechanism for the doctors by enabling them to avoid disclosure even when asked directly, clearly it also meant that it was extremely difficult for the patient who genuinely wanted to find out about his condition to obtain the information which he sought. Only by challenging the whole form of the communication, or, more specifically, the euphemistic terms in which it was constituted, or by otherwise rendering it inadequate for the doctors' purposes, could patients break out of this cycle.

The euphemistic mode of communication could be challenged successfully by persistent, or particularly pointed, demands for explicit information. Thus, the patient who persistently asked if he had cancer was likely to be told eventually. Through repeated requests for information the patient indicated that he did not accept that what he had been told was the whole truth and to have continued to respond to him in an evasively euphemistic way, when he was clearly dissatisfied with that sort of response, could have seriously undermined his trust in the doctor. But, even then, there was a reluctance to disclose. The very fact that a patient continued to petition for information might be interpreted as indicating that he was particularly agitated and worried and might not therefore be a suitable case for telling. Nevertheless, in the face of repeated demands, the pressures to disclose were such that this perception normally led only to delay in rendering the diagnosis rather than to its being withheld indefinitely.

Patients' attempts to find out about their condition proved to be particularly effective if accompanied by an appeal for 'the truth'. Such an appeal ('Is that the truth now?' or 'Honest?') was especially successful in eliciting a frank response not so much because it convinced the doctor of the patient's resolve, but rather because it left him with no alternative short of lying. And, of course, lying was strenuously avoided by the doctors because untruths, unlike semi-truths, could rebound on them later with disasterous consequences for the patient's confidence in them. Whereas half-truths could, if necessary, be built upon at a later date, lies could not. A demand for the truth immediately put the doctor's integrity on trial. Any prevarication in response to it would have amounted to a lie. There was, therefore, no way of responding honestly to such a request other than by giving a frank reply. However, patients were not simply told bluntly, 'Yes, you have cancer.' The news was always qualified by an accompanying statement stressing the more hopeful aspects of their condition.

> Yes, but it's treatable and we should be able to cure it. I wouldn't worry about it. There are many women going around without a breast you know.

> Well yes, I suppose you could call it a cancer. But this doesn't mean that you should worry about it. It's a curable kind. We have removed it all and we expect you to have no more trouble. So I don't think you have any cause to worry about it.

Very occasionally, a patient might also be able to obtain his prognosis. Although it was not observed during the study, apparently patients might sometimes ask whether they would survive their illness. In the interviews I was able to obtain some information on how the doctors might manage such requests. If the prognosis was thought to be good or, at least, if it was not certain that it was bad, the doctor's response to such an enquiry was relatively unproblematic. He would simply tell the patient that the outlook was thought to be good. Where the prognosis was considered to be unfavourable, only in exceptional circumstances would this be divulged to the patient. It was felt that a prediction of death would be too harrowing. However, on certain occasions the doctors did feel obliged to give some assessment. The main consideration appeared to be not whether the patient genuinely wanted to know or could take the news but rather the extent of his commitments, particularly if these commitments were invoked by the patient himself. It was generally agreed that such patients should be given the opportunity for making necessary arrangements.

> Occasionally you get someone who says, 'Have I got cancer? I must know because I've got a shop. . . .'Or, 'I've got an insurance policy or business interests which I must get settled up.' In that case you just have to tell them. And, very occasionally, they ask what their prognosis is and again, under those circumstances, you have to tell them. I mean, it would be terrible to tell someone, 'Oh yes, you'll be all right. You'll be fine', knowing perfectly well that they'll be dead in six months.

There was one other occasion on which the doctor might have to tell the patient what he had. The euphemistic form of communication often became inadequate for achievement of the doctors' objectives when patients refused to accept treatment. In such cases, because it failed to sufficiently alert patients to the gravity of their situation and the necessity for treatment, this mode of communication was a positive hindrance. Thus, while refusal of treatment was extremely rare, under these circumstances the doctor might again be forced to become more explicit in his communication, this time in order to acquire the patient's co-operation in treatment. Even then, he would at first attempt to impress the seriousness of his condition, and the need for treatment of it, upon the patient without recourse to 'cancer': 'This could be a danger to your life if it isn't treated.' This was usually sufficient to secure their co-operation. Only as a last resort would be patient be told explicitly that he had a malignancy. One of the doctors recounted the following tale.

> Give them every chance, apply considerable pressure, use all these vague terms. I'd one patient recently who went through all these stages . . . he had cancer of his penis. And, in the end I said, 'Do you know what this is?' And he said 'No'. I told him, 'This is cancer of the penis. It's going to get bigger, it's going to obstruct your water, it's going to get painful and it's going to spread to the glands. And yet, if you just come in and have it operated on, your chances of cure are 99 per cent. And he said, 'All right, I'll come in.' And he had the op. . .[1]

So, there were two occasions on which the euphemistic form of communication embodied in the routines might have to be discarded and replaced by disclosure: if the patient was particularly determined in his demand for explicit information or if he exhibited reluctance to undergo treatment. A patient with considerable commitments might also be given his prognosis if he requested it. However, as these occurrences were comparatively rare, clearly very few patients obtained their diagnosis and only a very tiny number were given their prognosis.

The Use of Uncertainty

One further aspect of the management of communication merits more detailed consideration in its own right. A central feature of the routines was the way in which professions of certainty or uncertainty were used in the management of communication and to limit the degree of disclosure to patients. For example, we have already seen how, even after clinical certainly had been established, the doctor would often use a pretence of uncertainty about the nature of the patient's condition as a device for avoiding disclosure to him. Davis (1966) introduced the concept of functional uncertainty to denote the practice of using a profession of uncertainty in this way and examined in some detail the way in which it served in the management of interaction with patients. However, in the present context, functional uncertainty did not consist of the doctors professing outright that they were uncertain. Once they had received the results of their investigations, they did not tell the patient, 'We do not know what you've got', or 'We're uncertain what the diagnosis is.' The use of uncertainty was more subtle than that. Rather, it was observed, the doctors would use an altogether different kind of terminology. The patient's condition was usually described by means of euphemisms such as 'suspicious cells', 'nasty cells', 'activity', 'might have become dangerous', and so on. While uncertainty is implied directly in terms like '*suspicious* cells' and, 'it *might* have become dangerous', other euphemisms, like 'activity' and 'nasty cells', might at first appear to contain no element of uncertainty. However, although terms like 'activity' and 'nasty cells' do not in themselves imply uncertainty, the fact that they are used instead of a specific diagnostic label, such as 'cancer', does imply that the doctor is sufficiently uncertain of the true nature of the condition to be unable to put a more precise label to it. In effect, when using these terms, he is saying to the patient, 'There were certainly some nasty cells and activity there but the condition was so ambiguous that I cannot put a name to it.' We see, then, that professions of uncertainty could come in two different guises. It was inherent in terms like 'suspicious cells' and present by default in euphemisms like 'activity' and 'nasty cells'. In either case, uncertainty was alluded to, not professed openly.

The use of this sort of terminology also solved a potential dilemma for the doctor: namely, how could he use a pretence of uncertainty to restrict information while at the same time conveying to the patient that he knew what he was doing? The method adopted was, as we have seen, to use terms which, while implying uncertainty in sufficient degree to allay patient fears, also avoided a more explicit profession of it. The doctors could not openly profess to be uncertain about the diagnosis after having completed their investigations without the risk of losing the patient's confidence in their ability to treat them. But, the use of terms like 'suspicious cells' displayed the appropriate combination of uncertainty and confidence in what they were doing to convince the patient that, while they might not be certain of the precise nature of their condition, they were sufficiently conversant with it to be able to treat it effectively. That is, the doctors attempted to convey to the pat-ient that, irrespective of whether they were certain of the exact nature of his condition, they were absolutely certain of their ability to treat it. Uncertainty over the diagnosis was always tempered by certainty over the method, and efficacy, of the treatment to be employed. The euphe-mistic mode of communication employed by the doctors fulfilled yet another function: it enabled them to tell patients as much of the truth as was consistent with the retention of hope, without lying to them.

In the employment of functional uncertainty diagnosis and prognosis were connected insofar as hope of a good prognosis was contained with-in uncertainty over the diagnosis. That is, the fact that the doctor was not certain of the exact nature of the condition implied that it could not be a very bad one. After all, a bad cancer would be easily diagnosed. However, the implications of the use of uncertainty in relation to the outlook were rather different from those involved in its use in connect-ion with the diagnosis. A profession of uncertainty about the prognosis could have the opposite effect upon the patient from a profession of uncertainty about the diagnosis. The doctor's uncertainty over the diagnosis could be interpreted as meaning that the condition might not be too bad. On the other hand, uncertainty over the prognosis could be interpreted as meaning that it might not be very good. As patients would expect that, if the doctor were certain that the prognosis was good, he would tell them so, for him to appear uncertain of it could indicate that the outlook was probably unfavourable. In this sense, uncertainty was functional with the diagnosis but could be dysfunction-al if applied to the prognosis. So, if asked for information relating to the prognosis, the doctor attempted to avoid giving the impression that he was uncertain. In order to give the patient hope over the prognosis he had to get as close to stating that he was certain of it as he possibly could. So, in many cases we saw a tendency towards something akin to a kind of functional *certainty* being employed where the prognosis was involved.[2] The different approaches to the use of uncertainty with the diagnosis and prognosis can be summarised as follows: because the ef-fects of professing uncertainty were opposite in the two cases, with the diagnosis the doctor had a tendency to maximise it while with the prog-nosis the tendency was to minimise it.

As we saw earlier, the extent to which the doctor could profess to be certain about the outlook depended upon his perception of the sever-ity of the patient's condition. If the doctor was almost sure that the patient was cured or if he believed that he would be free from the dis-ease for several years he would give him an unequivocally good prognosis. In other words, in cases where the doctor considered that it was relatively unlikely that such a positive statement would rebound on him, he saw no point in giving the patient cause for doubt and concern by portraying the prognosis as being anything less than certain. On the other hand, however, if the condition was more serious and the doctor had less reason to expect a favourable outcome or if, indeed, he believed the outlook to be hopeless, his assessment of the prognosis, while formulated in such a way as to imply a hopeful outlook, would also contain a trace of uncertainty. Although the doctor was aware of the impact a profession of uncertainty could have on the patient, he had to introduce it in some measure in order to avoid subsequent accusations of incompetence or deceit. But, given that the doctor sought to reassure the patient, when he professed to be uncertain about the prognosis he had to be careful how he did so. He had to strike a delicate balance between covering himself against possible future developments and not giving the patient cause for alarm. He attempted to achieve this by giving the patient the impression that he was *practically* certain without giving him to believe that he was *absolutely* certain.

> Patient: Did you get it all?
> Dr Craib: Almost certainly. Almost certainly. There's nothing for
>   you to worry about.

In this way, the doctor was able to give the patient as reassuring an assessment as possible while, at the same time, not committing himself, as one doctor said, 'to the fact that you have got everything when you may know very well you haven't.'

Summary and Appraisal

It is appropriate at this point briefly to summarise the argument of the last three chapters. The difficult nature of the problem which the doctors faced should not be underestimated. They had an extremely difficult type of interaction to cope with and were very anxious to ensure that no trouble resulted from it. While they believed that the great majority of patients did not want to know and would not react well to receiving either their diagnosis or an unfavourable prognosis, they also held the view that some patients could and should be told. The problem was that they had no way of ascertaining, with any certainty, whether patients genuinely wanted to know or how they would respond to disclosure. In response to these uncertainties they adopted the only safe course of action open to them: they avoided disclosure to all patients.

This provided a way of coping with uncertainty over patients' desire for information and probable reactions to being told that was consistent with the belief that most patients did not want to know and would not react well. Communication was also routinized. This ensured consistency in what patients were told, obviated the necessity of making decisions in individual cases, and avoided conflict over telling between members of the medical staff. As we saw, most of the time the routines succeeded in their objective of not revealing the nature and severity of their condition to patients. Only in the exceptional case, where the patient either continued to demand information or where he refused treatment, might the euphemistic form of communication enshrined in these routines be successfully overthrown and replaced by disclosure.

Now, it could be argued that there might have been another reason for the doctors not telling. Quite simply, they may have wished to avoid the unpleasant task of disclosure. No doctor likes to be the bearer of bad news. It is threatening to the patient and may carry an implication of failure on their part. It is always easier to give hope than to be brutally frank. The policy which the doctors pursued was, of course, entirely consistent with the implementation of such a desire. It could therefore be postulated that the doctors' expressed philosophy, which was dominated by the belief that the majority of patients did not want to know and could not stand to be told, was simply a way of justifying a policy which was actually a product of other, more personal, concerns. In short, the doctors might have wished to avoid the difficult task of informing a patient that he had cancer, or that the prognosis was poor, and might have sought refuge in a policy of not telling, using as justification for that policy the belief that disclosure would be detrimental to the majority of patients. If this were so, then the philosophy which they espoused, which was, after all, largely based upon assumptions, was merely an account (Scott and Lyman 1970) or convenient rationalisation for a policy to which they had become committed for other reasons. However, on balance, I consider it rather unlikely that a personal reluctance to disclose was central to the doctors' communication practices. The doctors maintained that their fundamental belief that the patient had the right to know, providing he wanted to and this would not be detrimental to him, transcended such personal considerations. Although it could not be established conclusively, there was no reason to believe that this view was not both valid and genuinely held. Moreover, implementation of the view that some patients should be told and the experience of disclosure as an unpleasant task are not mutually exclusive. People will often carry out tasks which they perceive as being distasteful in the performance of what they consider to be their duty. The doctors in the present study would probably have been prepared to tell had they been sure that the circumstances were right. Certainly the act of disclosure itself did not seem to hold any great fears for them. But, of course, they were only prepared to tell in those cases in which a bad reaction was considered to be extremely unlikely. Whereas disclosing to patients who were not suitable candidates for telling could certainly have been quite traumatic, with patients who could be counted upon to accept the news stoically, disclosure was not likely to be nearly so distressing. In addition, the doctors had a number of techniques for softening or mitigating the impact of disclosure on patients and, consequentially, minimising any discomfort which they themselves might have experienced in carrying out the task. They would always place the most optimistic interpretation on the patient's condition and only in exceptional circumstances would they admit that the disease had got beyond them. Thus, even on those occasions on which they had to tell, and where they were not at all sure of how the patient would react, disclosure appeared to be accomplished without too much discomfort on the doctors' part.

For the moment, this concludes discussion of the methods of communication employed by the doctors. The operation of these practices is represented in more dynamic form in subsequent chapters where case histories are presented. Chapter 5 examines the role of the nurses in the communication process.

Notes

1. In the exceptional case, even that degree of explicitness may not achieve its objective. This doctor went on to describe a similar case. '. . . Oddly enough, another one was a young man who also had cancer of the penis . . . which, when you think that we see one or two every three years, is rather extraordinary . . . who flatly refused. He was Mr Donald's patient and he told him what it was and what would happen. He again refused. He was a young chap and this was the final indignity—to have his penis cut off . . . he refused, yes. He'd rather die than have it cut off. And he did.'

2. Davis (1966) uses the term 'dissimulation' to denote this practice of rendering a prognosis, which is not substantiated clinically, as if it were certain. However, in the present context the doctors were not guilty of outright deceit. They had some justification for professing certainty in those cases in which they did so. This was only done where, as far as they knew, the outlook could be good. Certainly, in those cases, they did not know for sure that it would be bad.

5 THE NURSES

We have seen how the doctors managed interaction with patients and attempted to control their awareness. However, the nursing staff also occupied a central position within the communication network. They were constantly engaged in interaction with patients and were in a position, had they wished, to bring the doctors' efforts at communication management to nought. As we shall see, for a number of reasons this did not happen. Certainly, the nursing staff were usually in possession of the sort of information which the patient might wish to obtain. They were all agreed that they were kept well informed about the patient's diagnosis and treatment. Information about changes in these was passed on to them at reporting sessions which took place at the beginning of each shift. More detailed information about patients' conditions was obtained by more senior members of the nursing staff (Sisters and, occasionally, Staff Nurses) who attended the weekly ward conferences. Much of this was also passed on to the rest of the staff. Clearly the nursing staff were potentially a very important source of information. What were their perspectives on telling, what did they communicate to patients and how did they manage interaction with them?

The Nurses' Perspective

The nurses knew that the doctors had a conservative approach to informing patients about their condition and that the diagnosis and prognosis would be withheld unless it was absolutely necessary to disclose them. They shared the doctors' perspective on telling and wholly endorsed the policy of not volunteering the diagnosis and prognosis. 'I think the doctors tell them as much as is necessary for the patient to know. I don't think they should be told they've got cancer. I don't think patients should be told unless absolutely necessary.'

None of the nurses advocated a policy of routinely informing all patients. This harmony of perspectives effectively obviated the emergence of conflict between the medical and nursing staff over what patients should be told.

The nurses advanced the same reasons for not telling patients as the doctors. Principally, they believed that patients did not want to know.

I don't think they want to know. I don't think they want it put into words. As long as they just suspect. . . I think I'd feel a bit like that myself. I would know from the treatment what it was but, as long as nobody said it, I would still have a bit of hope.

They did concede, though, that some patients would probably like to be told but they were assessed to be very much in the minority. 'I have no doubt that most patients are frightened to know the truth. But, of course, a few of them *would* like to know.'

However, while they believed that the great majority of patients did not want to know, they also felt, like the doctors, that a large proportion of them were probably aware that they had a malignancy. This conclusion was partly based upon remarks passed by patients and certain 'hints' which they dropped.

They'll never say, 'We know what's wrong with us', but they'll drop a hint, 'I'm going to make the most of my life once I'm out of this place.' The other day I was doing a patient's dressing and said, 'Oh, this is just a little thing.' 'Oh no,' she said, 'Nurse, it's not a pimple, it's not a boil, but *you'll* know what it is.' And she knew that she had cancer.

In some cases, the assessment that patients were aware was founded upon what would appear to be rather flimsy evidence.

JM: How do you know they know?
Nurse C: Well you just do. It's sort of instinct more than anything else. You can really tell. If you think a patient's worried, that's a tell-tale sign although they don't say anything.

Mostly, though, the nurses simply assumed that patients *must* be aware.

They must know. I think anybody who's intelligent enough will know. For instance, radium's widely broadcast now. So there's not many people don't know when they're getting radiotherapy what it's for.

If women have a breast off it's well known that the only reason you take the whole breast off is if you've got cancer. Also, if they do a bilateral adrenalectomy plus an oopherectomy, which is massive abdominal surgery, they're bound to know.

But while they felt that patients were probably aware, or at least suspected, that they had a malignancy, the nurses did not believe that they wished to have it confirmed. The absence of confirmation would leave them with hope. In this, of course, they were in accord with the views of the medical staff. To some extent, this orientation reflected what the nurses believed they themselves would like to know should they ever be in a similar position.

> Well, I personally don't think I'd like to be told. I think that if I had a malignant disease, I'd rather not be told because I'd feel there's no bettering in it. There's treatment, but there's no cure. I could always hope I might not have it although I was almost one hundred percent sure that I did.

If, as the nurses believed, most patients preferred not to know, to have given them their diagnosis or prognosis would have been to have invited a bad reaction from them. This prospect was certainly a major factor in determining the nurses' attitudes towards telling. While they acknowledged that some patients would react well, or eventually come to terms with the knowledge, the majority, they believed, would take the news very badly.

> I don't think most of them are emotionally fit to cope with it. I'm sure they would get quite hysterical about it. Especially the ones that have heard a lot about cancer and think it's a killer and that's it.

> They would just break down. Some would just shut up and go into a shell. They won't speak, won't eat and won't drink and just lose the will to live generally.

However, it was not simply that disclosure would cause patients distress: the nurses also feared that distressed and agitated patients would make life more difficult for them. 'I think the atmosphere in the ward would be worse if they were told. And I think it would make it worse for us. I think it would make them very difficult.'

While the nurses believed that patients in general would not benefit from disclosure, most of them felt that certain patients should be told. They differed in the extent to which they did so. Some nurses were more in favour of telling than others. Their comments upon which patients should be told ranged from, 'I think quite a lot of them should be told', to 'I don't think there's any reason why anybody should be told'. Those nurses who would have liked to have known themselves were likely to be more disposed towards telling. However, none of the nurses advocated giving patients their prognosis. The main indication for telling, in the nurses' view, was if a patient asked outright. 'Those who have an idea what's wrong and ask the consultant point blank, then they should be told as gently as possible. If it is somebody quite intelligent who said, "I want to know". I think they should be told.'

Some of them even expressed the view that the patient who asked had a *right* to know. 'Well, I think that if they ask to be told the truth, then they definitely should. After all, it's their life and it's their body we're chopping up.'

Among the other types of patient whom they felt should be told were, 'a young man who has to provide for a family', or, 'a businessman (who) usually wants to know the truth to put his affairs in order and check his will'. But, even then, they would usually only be in favour of telling if they enquired. Moreover, while maintaining that certain categories of patient should be informed, they qualified it by saying that this should only be done if one could be sure that their reaction to disclosure would not be an adverse one: 'If he was capable of knowing', 'if he can be told', 'as long as they're not the neurotic type'. One had also to be sure that the patient genuinely wanted to know. But, how could they be sure of those questions? The problem was that they could not. The nurses were aware of this.

> But, you see, how are we to *know* who to tell and who not to tell. It's so difficult and you can make a mistake, a bad one, by telling somebody who'll crack up.

> Some would probably accept it. Some would prefer to be told. But it's a big decision to make. You don't really know.

Certainly, the fact that a patient asked could not be taken as evidence that they wanted to know the truth or that they could 'take it'.

> Some of them who ask and say, 'I definitely want to know', are the ones who go to pieces when they're told.

> I've known a businessman who wanted to put his affairs in order and asked the doctors for the truth and died of shock from a coronary thrombosis.

While acknowledging the problem the nurses offered no solution to it except that one had to 'play it by ear'. But nor was it necessary for them to have a solution to the dilemma. The nurses did not tell the patients. Even if they believed that a patient should be told, they would not undertake to do so. None of the nurses, even those with long experience in the treatment of cancer patients, admitted to ever having told a patient that he had cancer. Certainly none did so during the course of the study. Telling was acknowledged to be the doctors' prerogative.[1]

Well I can't. Sometimes you wish you could tell them because they are wanting to know. But a nurse has to just go and tell the doctor that they want to know. It's stipulated in the rules that we don't tell.

But a nurse can't tell them if they've got it even if they ask, because they're not allowed to. It's the doctor's responsibility.

So, in addition to sharing the doctors' perspective on telling and thereby believing that most patients should not be told, even where they felt that a particular patient should be informed, the nurses did not consider that it was their place to do so. In view of that, how then, did they manage patients' enquiries?

Management of Communication

Only very seldom were the nurses asked explicitly by patients if they had cancer. The great majority had *never* been asked that question. Those who had been asked, even when they had worked on Ward 4C for a number of years, had only come across it once or twice. It was even more unusual for them to be asked outright for a prognosis. Indeed, it was comparatively rare for patients to question nurses about their diagnosis and prognosis at all,[2] that is, even by means of more indirect questions such as, 'What's wrong?' or 'Am I clear?' Although some of the nurses were under the impression that they were questioned most often, 'They probably ask the nurses more because they find them more approachable', patients were much more likely to address those questions to the doctors. This does not, of course, mean that the nurses were never asked questions relating to the nature and severity of patients' conditions. They were. It was simply that they encountered them less frequently than the doctors. Much more common was for patients to question the nurses about their treatment. 'They don't ask what they've got. They ask questions about the treatment or the tablets.'

In this respect the nurses probably faced more enquiries than the doctors.

There was some dispute among the nurses as to which sector of the nursing staff was questioned most often. The junior nurses were evenly divided.

> I think they ask the junior nurses most because they're working with them more and get to know them better. I think they're frightened of authority a lot of them. Junior nurses give them their tea and coffee and chat away to them but Sister does the ward rounds. So she's almost in comparison with the doctor and they don't like to chat so easily with her.

> I think it's more the senior staff they ask that sort of thing. They haven't asked me what's wrong. Because they're scared how it might affect me I think. They worry about how it might affect a young nurse.

On the other hand, most, but not all, of the senior nurses believed that they were the prime target for questions. While it was difficult to gauge with any accuracy, the distribution of questions about the diagnosis and prognosis did, in fact, appear to be biased towards them. However, *any* nurse could be questioned about these matters. How did they handle it when they were?

The most common method employed for managing patients' questions, particularly by the more junior nurses, was to refer the enquiring patient to a senior nurse or a doctor.[3]

> Miss Stephen: What's this thing on my leg nurse?
> Nurse F: I don't know. The doctors would be the best persons to ask that. Would you like me to get one of them to speak to you?

Alternatively, the junior nurses might avoid having to answer a question by making some excuse and absenting themselves from the patient. 'Well, you just say you've got something to do. "Oh, I'm busy. I'll come back later." They drop it. You just say, "Well, I've got to give something to Staff Nurse", or something like that and you just get away from it.'

Enquiries were handled differently according to the seniority of the nurse who encountered them. Senior nurses were much more likely to answer questions themselves. To an extent, this was because they often had little choice. They could not plead ignorance about a patient's con-

dition as plausibly as a junior nurse could. A Sister or Staff Nurse would
be expected to know the diagnosis and at least to have a good idea of
the prognosis. More importantly, though, they usually felt equipped to
answer patients' queries while the junior nurses often did not. The senior nurses knew what to say. They had become conversant with what to
tell patients by observing the ways in which the doctors managed communication with them. 'I suppose I just started my way through listen-
ing to the consultants. You watch what the doctors say to the patients
and the techniques they use and do the same.'

The junior nurses had much less experience of what the medical staff
told patients, primarily because they often lacked the opportunity to
acquire it. 'I haven't been round with the doctors so I don't really know
what they say.' 'I'm not there when they're telling them.' They were,
therefore, much less likely to take it upon themselves to reply to patients'
questions. However, this does not mean that the junior nurses never
undertook to do so. Whether they did or not depended in part upon
their awareness of what were considered to be the appropriate responses. This, in turn, was a product of the extent to which they had been
able to observe the doctors' methods of managing communication with
patients.

However, if telling had been based upon assessment of individual
cases, it is doubtful whether even the senior and experienced members
of the nursing staff would have felt as confident in responding to
questions. The fact that communication was routinized was crucial
in affording nurses the freedom to do so. They were aware that the
doctors' communication to patients was of a routine nature.

> I think they have a basic thing that everybody says. Some may go
> into a little more detail and have a better manner of putting it
> across, but basically it's much the same. They tell them the same
> type of thing—give them the same answers.

Moreover, they were also able to articulate those set procedures for
telling and knew where to apply them.

> For cancer of the breast it's always the same. They explain it in
> the same way. 'We'll take you to theatre and examine the lump
> under the microscope and, if we think it's anything suspicious,'—
> you probably know the routine—'we'll remove the breast in case
> it gives you any trouble in the future.'

They did not, therefore, have to make decisions in individual cases. Nor did they need to know what the doctor had told a particular patient. They knew which routines pertained to which types of case at particular stages of treatment. They simply had to implement them. The routinized nature of communication virtually eliminated the risk of nurses communicating something which was at variance with what the patient might be told by a member of the medical staff.

Patients asked the nurses the same questions about their diagnosis as they asked the doctors: What is it? What did they find? What caused this? What was that lump? — and so on. They received the same replies. Questions posed by patients before their operation or prior to the completion of investigations were relatively easily managed by the nurses. They simply told them that their questions could not be answered at that stage.

> Mr Wyatt: What is this thing nurse?
> Nurse P: Well, we won't know till you come back from theatre. We'll have to wait till we get all your X-rays and reports and things together. But there's something not quite right at the back of your tongue and Mr Moorehead's going to take you to theatre tomorrow and he's going to look and see what it is. He'll let you know then.

Questions about the diagnosis were more likely to be asked after investigations were completed. At that stage, a definite answer was required. I observed no examples of nurses being asked the direct question, 'Have I got cancer?' However, according to them, on the rare occasions when it was posed, and where they did not refer the question to a member of the medical staff, they would respond to it in the same vein as the doctors. 'One or two might ask, "Have I got cancer?" But we just waffle round it by saying, "If it had been left it might have become one." The same sort of things that the doctors say.'

Questions about the diagnosis which did not make explicit reference to cancer were more common. Again, the appropriate routine response was implemented.

> Mrs Kay: What sort of lump was it Sister?' (radical mastectomy)
> Sister S: Well, there were some suspicious cells in it and if it had been left much longer it would have turned nasty. The doctor had to take away a little more just to make absolutely sure that

they got away the whole bit.

Questions pertaining to the patient's symptoms were managed by giving a plausible answer which did not refer to their underlying cause.

> JM: If somebody with a bronchial cancer says, 'Why can't I breathe? or 'Why am I coughing so much?'
> Nurse L: Because you've got so much sputum in there that you need to get it up and the more you cough the better.

It was extremely rare for patients to ask the nurses questions relating to their prognosis, however, when they did, the nurses' replies were again consistent with the routine responses employed by the doctors.

> Mr Gibson: Did they get it all do you think nurse?
> Nurse J: Oh yes. I think so. That's why they took so much away— to make sure that they did. I don't think you've got anything to worry about.

> Mr Smith: Sister, I was wondering, do you think I'll have to come back in?
> Sister W: Oh no. I shouldn't think so. We certainly don't expect you to have to.

When answering these questions, the nurse might also refer the patient to the doctor or a senior member of the nursing staff.

> Mrs Lane: Is that me all clear now?
> Nurse K: As far as I know, yes. But you'd better ask the Sister or the doctor.

Questions about the purpose of treatment, which were more frequently encountered, were answered without mentioning the diagnosis.

> Mr Royle: What's the radiotherapy for nurse?
> Nurse H: Well, it's to get rid of that swelling. You'll feel much better when the treatment's finished.

Additional or supplementary treatment was explained in terms of making sure: 'In case there are any cells lying about—to kill them off.'

The role played by the nursing staff in the communication network can be summarised as follows. They shared the doctors' perspective on telling, believing that, by and large, it would be wrong to disclose to patients. They did not, therefore, divulge the diagnosis or prognosis. Even in those cases where they felt that a particular patient should be told they would not do so, believing that this was the sole prerogative of the medical staff. While it was comparatively rare for the nurses to face questions concerning the patient's diagnosis and prognosis, when they did encounter them, and offered a reply, their answers were consistent with the routine responses utilised by the doctors.

Having examined how both the medical and nursing staff manipulated the communication process in order to manage patients' awareness, in the following chapters I consider the other side of the interaction: how the patients managed uncertainty, in terms of their desire for information and their efforts to acquire it, and the ways in which they attempted to manipulate the communication network for their own ends.

Notes

1. This supports the findings of other workers (Freidson 1970, 141; Coser 1962, 75; Davis 1963, 59) that nurses do not disclose to patients. An exception to this is Glaser and Strauss's finding that 'sometimes nurses will wittingly break the institutional rule that only the doctor may disclose dying to the patient' ('Temporal Aspects of Dying as a Non-Scheduled Status Passage', *Am. J. Sociol*, 1965, p. 54).
2. This contrasts strongly with Glaser and Strauss's finding (1965, p. 45) that, when the information received from the medical staff is limited or incomplete, the burden of coping with patients' questions falls upon the nurses.
3. Sudnow (1967, p. 117) and Quint (1965, p. 123) found this tactic to be the most common way of handling questions from dying patients.

6 AWARENESS AND DESIRE FOR INFORMATION

The previous chapters set out what patients were told in different contexts and attempted to analyze and explain those communication practices. I now consider the patients themselves. Patients adjusted to their illness in very different ways in terms of desire for information and the ways in which it was sought. The next five chapters undertake a detailed description and analysis of those different patterns of adaptation. I begin in this chapter by examining patients' awareness and desire for information upon entering the ward: how much did they know about their condition, how had they become aware and how much did they want to know and why? As we will see, some patients wanted and sought additional information while others did not. Chapter 7 documents the careers of patients who did not want to know. The following chapters examine the ways in which information was sought and obtained by those who wanted to find out about their condition. The different patterns of adaptation are conceived of as different ways of responding to uncertainty.

Several different types of patient career were identified in terms of differential awareness and desire for information. Patients' knowledge of their condition and desire for information was obtained in interviews while observation of their interactions with others supplied data on the implementation of their desires and the different patterns of adaptation to knowledge, or suspicion, of the nature of their condition, which they adopted. Patients were classified according to whether they knew or suspected upon admission to the ward. Their awareness, combined with their subsequent desire for further information and efforts to obtain it, provided the basis for their allocation to particular categories of patient career. But, of course, patients' awareness and desire for information did not always remain constant throughout their stay in hospital. The dynamic and changing nature of the careers within these relatively static categories will become evident shortly.

The presentation of the material on the patients posed something of a dilemma. While certain important features of patient adaptation had clearly to be examined in relatively discrete sections I also wanted to convey the processual, interactional and developmental nature of patients' responses to their illness and efforts either to augment their knowledge or to avoid realization and maintain hope. I have attempted to illustrate the dynamic quality of these processes by means of case histories. Accordingly, chapters 7 and 9 are given over almost entirely to outlining different types of patient career. There, typical cases are described and analyzed individually. The patients are identified by means of pseudonyms. Certain other of their characteristics have also been altered to render them unidentifiable.

In this chapter I attempt to quantify and explain the variety of responses and degrees of awareness which patients displayed towards their illness.[1]

Patients' Awareness

Nine separate categories of patient were identified in terms of their awareness and desire for information upon admission to the ward. These are represented in summary form in Table 1.

Table 1 Patients' Awareness and Desire for Information

Group	No. of patients	Awareness	Want Diagnosis	Want Prognosis
1	32	Suspected	No	No
2	9	Suspected	Yes	No
3	14	Knew	—	No
4	6	Suspected	Yes	Yes
5	3	Knew	—	Yes
6	1	Knew	—	—
7	6	Did not suspect		
8	3	Misled into believing that they did not have cancer		
9	6	Benign — diagnosis and prognosis unproblematic		

How much did the patients know about their condition? Of the 80 patients in the sample, six had benign conditions and are excluded from the following analysis. Of the remaining 74, 65 either knew or suspected that they had cancer on admission to the ward. Those who knew or suspected, therefore, constituted 88 per cent of the reduced sample. Only those patients who said unequivocally that they had cancer were classified as knowing. Those who merely displayed an awareness that they *might* have the disease: 'It might be cancer'; 'It's probably cancer'; 'I think it's cancer but I don't know for sure', were included in the suspicious category. As Table 1 shows, of the 65 patients who knew or suspected that they had cancer, 47 only *suspected* that this is what they had. Therefore, only 28 per cent, or about a quarter, of the patients who knew or suspected, actually *knew,* or rather said they knew, that they had the disease. The nine patients who did not know or suspect (Groups 7 and 8) also included three who had suspected cancer at one time but had been informed by medical staff elsewhere that they did not have the disease. But for having been diverted, they would probably have retained their suspicion until their admission to the ward. Had they done so, the proportion of those knowing or suspecting would have risen to 92 per cent. However, for present purposes, namely an assessment of patients' awareness upon admission to the ward, they are classified as not knowing or suspecting. As for the other six patients who did not appear to know or suspect, it was not possible to establish conclusively whether they knew or not. While they did not *indicate* any knowledge or suspicion of the nature of their condition, some of them may well have suspected or known.

The great majority of patients had, then, at least a suspicion that they might have a malignancy on admission to the ward.[2] How did they come to know or suspect? Their initial awareness was derived from a variety of sources, the most important of which was their own perception of their symptoms. Most patients associated a lump, or a sore that would not heal, with the possibility of malignancy: 'You always think of cancer when you've got a lump. . . ' In short, their suspicions were often a product of their own lay knowledge of the disease. This was especially so in the case of breast cancer patients and those with other palpable or visible lesions.[3] This probably reflected the importance of the visibility of symptoms in the process of becoming aware and the fact that certain types of symptomatology are more clearly identified with cancer by the lay public than are others. For example, patients with a breast lump are likely to be more immediately aware of the possibility of cancer than those with an internal disorder which might not be so readily associated with malignancy. However, as we will see, even for the latter, usually other clues would swiftly conspire to induce suspicion. Patients' awareness of the nature of the disease, for example the fact that it could recur or spread, was also often quite highly developed. They were even able, to some extent, to differentiate between more and less serious forms of it. The import of patients' lay knowledge was not confined to the process of self diagnosis and, as will become apparent, exerted a continuing influence upon their perceptions of their illness and reactions to it throughout their stay in hospital.

Friends, relatives and acquaintances who had had the disease themselves, or who knew someone who had, were another important source of information. Many patients compared their condition with that of

others whom they knew to have had cancer. In this way they often
deduced that their condition was probably the same. This comparison
might, or might not, involve actually discussing their fears with such a
key informant.

General practitioners did not volunteer the diagnosis to patients but,
if asked by them, they did occasionally help to confirm their suspicions.
Among the replies which patients received from GPs to the question,
'Is it cancer?' were, 'Well, it's a sort of cancer', or, 'Well it might be,
but I don't think it's a dangerous one', or, 'It's a possibility that
shouldn't be overlooked'. Of course, the patients must have suspected
before they asked that question.

The time taken to admit them to the ward was also subject to
interpretation by patients with a swift admission often being taken to
indicate that something serious was wrong.

> They got me in pretty quick. That'll be because they thought it
> might be cancer you see.

> With not having any pain or anything, I thought they dealt with
> me very quickly. I didn't think it was much but that really set me
> thinking it might be cancer.

On the other hand, if the patient felt that he had not been admitted
quickly, this was often interpreted by him as being a good sign.

> Well, the longer it goes on the more you wonder if they've forgotten
> you. Of course, the longer it goes on you think to yourself you
> can't be that ill.

> I feel that if it was malignant they would have had me in sooner, so I
> wasn't worried.

The perception of whether one was admitted quickly or not was
highly variable but, usually, being admitted within a fortnight of the outpatient consultation was taken to constitute just cause for alarm. A delay
of six weeks or more was a hopeful sign.

In the hospital there were other clues. The ward itself was fairly well
known as dealing mainly with cancer patients: 'Well, this is the cancer
ward isn't it?' Ward 4C was, of course, somewhat atypical in that, apart
from the gynaecology and dental patients, who were seen as being distinct, it dealt exclusively with malignancy and was fairly well known for

its specialty. Cancer patients on general surgical wards might not be so well clued in. However, the significance of the ward's atypicality should be put into perspective. By no means all patients were aware of its specialty and among those who were this was only one clue among many indicating the probable nature of their condition. In addition to the ward itself, one of the surgeons was especially well known as a specialist in malignant diseases: 'I've heard it's cancer he goes in for mostly. He's the cancer man', and many of the patients associated radiotherapy with the treatment of cancer. One or two said meaningfully that they had attended the 'Radiotherapy Department'. The sign at the entrance to the department read: 'Radio Therapy — Isotopes'.

The suspicion that they might have cancer usually prompted patients to consult their doctor but in other cases this fear led to delay. One woman had delayed reporting with a breast lump for eighteen months while another had tended a fungating breast mass by herself for two years.

I felt this lump but I didn't tell when I should have. To tell the truth, I was frightened. But, whenever I told my daughter, she got moving.

I thought about it (going to the doctor) but I just thought 'Oh no.' I was terrified. I couldn't think about it.

One patient had seen no point in consulting with cancer. 'I had made up my mind that it was cancer you see, and they say it's incurable, so there was no point in doing anything.'

Delay was often associated with attempts to deny that they had cancer, to define the condition as non-serious, or to otherwise explain it away. One patient clung to the hope that her condition was simply something which had developed through playing badminton, another maintained the belief that his 'false teeth had brought on an ulcer', while still others erected other explanations.

I just said it came from the thrombosis in my leg. That was my idea.

I had a slight discharge from the breast and some soreness. I thought it might be one of the little things that happens when the menopause starts. I hoped that was all it was.

Patients often maintained such conceptions of their condition for long periods and only consulted eventually when 'forced' to do so either by the worsening of their condition or through pressure from others.

> I'm bothered a lot with arthritis and put it down to that. But, when I began to *feel* the lump I went to the doctor. When it was just the pain I wasn't going to bother with it. And, of course, then my husband made me go.

However, some patients who were eventually forced to consult due to their worsening condition were able to maintain their alternative explanations after they were in hospital. This was especially true of a number of those who did not want to face the possibility that they could have cancer. For example, one woman suffering from low back pain and severe pain down both legs due to metastases from a previous breast cancer which she acknowledged was 'probably malignant' appeared to persist in the belief that she might have rheumatism.

> JM: Is the present trouble connected with your last admission?
> Mrs F: I don't think so. I hope not. It could be, but I don't think so. I think it might just be rheumatism.

A man who was readmitted with lung metastases, having suspected malignancy on his previous admission, attempted to neutralise the potential cue of being referred to the cancer specialist with a 'lung infection' in the following way. 'I suppose he referred me to Mr Moorhead because I'd been seeing him anyway for check-ups. I don't think it's got anything to do with my last thing.'

Even for those patients who did not delay, sometimes the suspicion of cancer was not, of itself, sufficient to induce them to consult their doctor. Some required, and sought, legitimation of their consultation from significant others. This was particularly so if the patient was not in pain or if the condition appeared to him to be minor. The fact that there was often no pain associated with the growth was an important factor in delay. Time and again patients said that the absence of pain had led them to believe that it could not be serious. 'It wasn't sore and you think, "Am I making a mountain out of a mole-hill?"' When it was required relatives always provided the necessary legitimation. 'It was my daughter that made me go. I wasn't sure it was worth bothering about so I asked her.'

Other patients required to be prodded into going to the doctor and the fact that a daughter or husband or other relative had made them go was mentioned frequently. 'I wasn't going to come but my wife said that it could be cancer and that I must see about it.'

Some patients even invited and welcomed being persuaded.

I knew that when I showed it to my husband he would make me go. I couldn't bring myself to go on my own.

Well, I thought that if I boasted to as many people as possible that I was going to the doctor, it would force me to go.

Irrespective of their manoeuvrings, all the patients eventually landed in hospital. Having outlined how they acquired their initial awareness, I now go on to examine how far, and for what reasons, they wanted to extend it, if at all, once they were there.

Desire for Information

For a number of the patients finding out about their condition did not appear to be an issue at all. Firstly there were six patients, three men and three women, who did not appear even to suspect that they might have cancer. Two of the men had lung cancer while the other had a rodent ulcer. The women's conditions were: Hodgkin's disease, an epithelioma on the base of the tongue, and continuing back pain following a mastectomy five years previously. I must emphasise that these patients did not *appear* to know or suspect that they had a malignancy. Some of them may well have suspected or known and it could simply be that I was unable to ascertain the nature and extent of their awareness. Nevertheless, none of them sought to obtain a diagnosis or to acquire information on the outlook for their condition. They appeared to be perfectly satisfied with the diagnosis which they had been given and with the doctors' assurances, sometimes implicit, that all would be well. Mr Douglas was satisfied that he had an ulcer which would not bother him again. In that he was correct. His rodent ulcer would not return. For Mrs Page, the removal of 'a hard bit' on her tongue was unproblematic and Miss Wright, once spinal metastases had been found, did not query that she had 'a softening of her bones' which would 'be set to rights by X-ray treatment'. Mrs Martin, who had Hodgkin's disease, did not waver from the belief that the lump in her neck was 'due to some sort of infection', despite having a splenectomy. She saw nothing strange in having her spleen removed in order to treat the cause of the lump. This she explained in terms of the infection emanating from her spleen.

> Mrs M: They took a lump out of my neck and tested it to see what treatment I would need. Then I had my spleen removed. They thought it had some connection with this thing in my neck. I suppose that's where the infection came from and now they've taken it away it should be OK.
> JM: So they've cured the infection now?
> Mrs M: Oh yes. I expect to be getting home soon.

The two men with lung cancer apparently accepted that they had a 'chest infection' and were receiving radiotherapy 'to clear it up'. Mr Gray came into the ward having been told by his GP that he had 'a patch of pneumonia in (his) chest'. In hospital, in response to communication from the consultant, this diagnosis was revised to 'an infection in my lung'. This did not alter his belief that his condition was a relatively simple one. 'Well, it's just an infection. He just said the radiotherapy would clear it up. I suppose that's all I needed to know—that it would clear it up. I don't think there's any problem.'

The possibility that they might have cancer did not seem to have occurred to any of these patients. They were entirely satisfied with the explanations which they had received. All six were discharged after treatment apparently believing that it had been successful and unproblematic and that they were cured. Only Mr Douglas, and possibly Mrs Page, were justified in their optimism.

Then there were the six patients who had benign conditions. There were two sorts of patient in this group: those who knew their condition was benign and those who had been told it most probably was benign. For the two patients who knew for certain that their condition was benign, there was no problem. The other four patients all had breast conditions and had all suspected cancer at one time.

> Well, a few weeks ago I had a soreness in my breast and examined it and found a lump. I wasn't going to go to the doctor but my husband said you couldn't be too careful. His father had cancer of the stomach you see.

However, they were informed that their condition was probably non-serious. This was occasionally done when they were first seen as an outpatient. The possibility that their condition might be serious was left open but played down.

> I'm pretty certain that this is just a simple thing but we'll take a bit of it out, just in case, and have a look at it under the microscope and, even if it looks as if it might become malignant, we'll remove the breast. But, as I say, I don't think it is, so I don't think it'll be necessary. But we'll take that thing away anyway.

This attempt at reassurance very largely succeeded in its objective. The patient's fears were kept to a minimum.

> Well, I'm not concerned because the doctor said he thought it wasn't serious. He said he was pretty sure it was something kind of tissue and that he would take it out. He said it wasn't really anything to worry about. So I'm not really worried about it although I suppose there is just a chance it could be cancer.

> No, I'm not really worried. He told me that he was 99 per cent certain that it wasn't anything malignant and you can't get much surer than that.

While their fears were not entirely dispelled, the relative possibilities had been presented to the patients in such a way as to reduce considerably the degree of apprehension which they might otherwise have experienced. The remnants of uncertainty were finally dispelled when it was confirmed that their condition was benign. This was swiftly communicated to them. All patients with benign tumours were informed categorically that their condition was harmless. This they accepted. During their stay in the ward, these patients did not ask questions about their diagnosis or prognosis because there was no point in doing so. The doctor's profession of uncertainty precluded questioning about the diagnosis which, when established and conveyed to the patient, meant that the prognosis became unproblematic. No patient with a benign condition was discharged believing that he had cancer.

The final group of patients for whom the nature of their condition was unproblematic were the three who had been misled into believing that they did not have cancer prior to their admission to Ward 4C. They were all readmissions. They had all suspected cancer at one time, and had apparently wanted to know, but in previous admissions to other wards had been given to believe that they did not have the disease. They were to maintain this belief for the duration of their stay in the ward. Because they had been misled into believing that they did not have a malignancy, their diagnosis and prognosis were unproblematic for them. They fully expected to get well. All three died. A brief description of two of these cases follows.

Mrs Falconer was a forty-one year old mother of two teenage sons. When I first saw her she detailed the history of her condition up to the time of her latest admission for radiotherapy to her spine. She was convinced that her condition was benign.

Mrs F: Well, it all started four years ago when I had a sort of tumour in my elbow which was removed. Then next year I had radiotherapy for a lump that came up in the armpit. That was the lymph gland.

JM: Was that a success?

Mrs F: At that time, yes. Then the following year I got an operation for more or less the same thing but that wasn't a success and they had to take the arm off.

JM: Was that successful?

Mrs F: Yes indeed.

JM: Why did they remove the arm?

Mrs F: Well, it was this tumour I'd had in my elbow I suppose.

JM: What are you in for now?

Mrs F: I was complaining of pain in the lumbar region and I was in a few weeks ago for radiotherapy to the lower region. I'm in for radiotherapy to the upper part now. It's a benign sort of thing that I have and fortunately it succumbs to radiotherapy. It's not a cancer, it's a benign thing that succumbs to radiotherapy when it gets worse again.

JM: One of the things I'm interested in is explanation to the patient — you know, keeping patients informed. Who told you it was benign?

Mrs F: The orthopaedic surgeon when I was in another ward. He told my husband the same thing a while ago. I was a bit impatient one day and asked if it was cancer. He took me into his office and explained about it. He said it was benign and that he knew a man who'd had the same as me for ten years and that it went the same way it came.

JM: So you were worried that it might have been cancer?

Mrs F: Of course, yes. I had thought that it was probably a malignancy.

JM: So, what you were told must have been a relief?

Mrs F: Oh yes. It was indeed.

While receiving her course of radiotherapy Mrs Falconer noticed a partial paralysis in her legs and, upon reporting it, promptly underwent an operation to her spine. She was greatly alarmed by the restriction of movement in her legs.

I was scared that the movement of my legs would go completely. As far as I can make out, a vertebra was touching a nerve which was affecting the legs—they separated them or something.

She then suffered from a period of chronic constipation which caused her considerable distress. However, she eventually regained movement in both her legs and her bowels much to her relief. This restored her confidence and on the day of her transfer to another hospital for 'convalescence' she still believed that her condition was benign and that she would eventually recover.

Mrs F: I had radiotherapy to start with then, when my legs went, I had an operation on the spine. Then I got another ten shots of radiotherapy to where the operation had been.

JM: What was the treatment for?

Mrs F: Well, it was this benign condition which I have and which keeps recurring. I was pleased with my legs moving and feeling the bowel moving.

JM: You think they were good signs?

Mrs F: Oh yes. I think that shows I'm on the mend. And the doctors say it's coming on quite well, but it's up to the body so that's all they can tell me.

JM: Any worries about it now?

Mrs F: No. I just content myself that it'll take a while.

So despite her clearly deteriorating condition, Mrs Falconer was able to maintain the belief that it was benign and that her treatment would ultimately culminate in a cure. It was just a matter of time and patience. Had she not been assured that her condition was benign, her orientation would doubtless have been very different. She died shortly afterwards.

Mr Booth, a thirty-two year old teacher, was admitted with an inoperable renal carcinoma. He had previously had a tumour removed from his thigh in another ward and had been informed there that it was non-malignant. The growth, which was in fact malignant, had originally been misdiagnosed as a lipoma. He had not been made aware of the revised diagnosis.

> Mr B: Well, I was in ward —. I had a lump in my thigh—a soft fatty
>   lump. It was benign—a lipoma. I had an operation there and they
>   took it away. When I found the lump at first I went to pieces.
> JM: Why was that?
> Mr B: I thought it was a cancer.
> JM: But they put your mind at rest?
> Mr B: Yes. They said it was just a fatty lump and that there was
>   nothing to worry about. They called it a lipoma.
> JM: What are you in for now?
> Mr B: Well, now they've found I've inflamation round the kidney.
>   At first they thought they would take out the kidney but decided
>   against it and cleaned round it and removed the inflamation instead.
>   Then they sent me here for radiotherapy but they decided against
>   that and put me on a course of tablets.
> JM: Are you worried about your kidney in the same way you were
>   worried about your leg?
> Mr B: Oh no. That's just an infection. But I was very worried about
>   my leg.
> JM: Are they connected in any way?
> Mr B: Well, as I understand it, the infection came from the leg.

During the course of his treatment, Mr Booth remained convinced
that he had 'inflamation' and did not appear to be at all concerned
about it although he was impatient to get home. He assumed that he
would get well. I recorded the following conversation with him after he
had been in the ward for a month.

> Mr B: I've been on tablets to remove the rest of the inflamation on
>   the kidney.
> JM: Have you asked about it at all?
> Mr B: No. The only thing I really wanted to know was how long it
>   was going to take. They can't say for sure.
> JM: Are you worried about it?
> Mr B: I don't think so. Sometimes I get depressed about it. I think I
>   expected the recovery to be quick but I've been told it'll take a
>   while. I just want to get out but I suppose I'll just have to wait.
>   Before he transferred me here the doctor warned me that it would
>   be a long slow process and that I mainly needed rest.

Although he was aware that the growth in his leg and the kidney trouble were related, having been told that the former was benign Mr Booth saw no reason to suspect that he might have cancer. He had accepted, reluctantly, that his treatment would be 'a long slow process' but, at least, it was a process towards recovery. He took eventual cure for granted, his only concern being to get out of hospital as soon as possible. He died in the ward.

While their diagnosis and prognosis were apparently not a matter of concern for a small number of patients, the nature and severity of their condition was potentially a very important issue for the others. How much did the 65 patients who knew or suspected that they had cancer want to find out about their condition? Firstly, how many of those who suspected wanted to know their diagnosis?

Table 2 Desire for Confirmation of their Diagnosis among Patients who Suspected that they had Cancer

	Wanted confirmation	Did not want confirmation	Total
No.	15	32	47
%	32	68	100

Table 2 shows that of the 47 patients who suspected their diagnosis, only fifteen would have liked confirmation of it. This means that 68 per cent of those who suspected did not want to know for sure. But, if we assume that those patients who knew that they had cancer (18) also *wanted* to know, and include them along with the 'suspicious' patients who wanted to know, then 33 out of 65, or about half the patients, wanted to know their diagnosis. However, this requires some qualification. For those patients who knew their diagnosis it did not constitute a problem in terms of finding out: they knew already. When we take them together with those who did not want confirmation of their suspicions, we find that 50 out of 65, or three quarters, *wished,* or *required,* no information on their diagnosis. So, it was only for a quarter of the patients that the diagnosis was problematic: that is, for those who suspected that they had cancer and wanted to know.

How many of the 65 patients who suspected or knew their diagnosis wanted to know what their prognosis was? Only one of them professed actually to know her prognosis on admission to the ward: she believed that she was going to die. Of the remaining 64 only nine, or 14 per cent, wanted information relating to the outlook. But, as we will see later, even then their desire for information about the outlook did not extend to wanting to know if they were going to die.

So, while the great majority of patients either knew or suspected that they had cancer, only a minority wished to augment that knowledge by either confirming their diagnosis or by finding out about their prognosis. Why did so many patients elect to suffer the uncertainty grounded in suspicion rather than establish what they had and what the outlook was? The key lies in the interface between the twin concepts of uncertainty and hope.

The proposition that patients would attempt to cope with uncertainty by seeking to find out about their condition presupposed that they would want to know what they had and what the outlook was likely to be. Many did not. They would rather suffer from uncertainty than know the truth. They did so because, for them, to suffer the uncertainty was preferable to the risk of losing their hope. Suspecting and knowing are entirely different things. So long as a patient did not *know*, he could always retain the hope that he might not have cancer. In other words, with uncertainty there was hope.[4] Those patients who did not seek a true assessment of their prognosis did so for the same reason that patients did not seek confirmation of their diagnosis. As long as they were uncertain, there was hope of a favourable outcome. It was precisely because they suspected that they might have cancer and/or that the prognosis might be bad that patients did not seek to obtain information about them. If they had not suspected they would have had no reason to fear what they might find out. There were numerous examples that patients would rather retain hope than know the truth.

> No, I wouldn't like to be told if it was (cancer) although I know it could be. I think I'd be terribly worried. I'd rather just wait and see and hope that it's OK.

> I think it's better not to know. It would only worry me if I did. I just hope that I'll be all right. I might not like what they could tell me.

> Yes. All that I wanted to know is that I didn't want to know if it was bad news. If it had been cancer I didn't want to know that. I just wanted to know if I was going to get well. I left it up to the doctors.

However, some of those patients who chose not to find out often suffered great conflict over whether or not to enquire. Because they would have liked to have known if they did *not* have the disease or that the prognosis was *good,* in not asking there was a risk that they might be denying themselves the opportunity of establishing that their fears were groundless. But, of course, while they wanted to know if the news was likely to be good, they did not want to receive bad news. They could not seek reassurance by asking without running the risk of having their worst fears confirmed. They might be told that they *did* have cancer or that the prognosis was *not* good. This prospect effectively discouraged them from enquiring.

> Well, it passes through your mind if it's clear—like a cancerous trouble. But I haven't asked them and they haven't said so far. I could ask the doctor I suppose. He could only say yes or no. But I'm probably better not to know. I just went along quite happy with the treatment.

The doctor could have said 'no' so this patient did not ask. The risk involved in asking was accentuated because the patients usually believed that, if they asked, they would be told the truth: if they had cancer, the doctor would tell them so. Given their assumption that their enquiry would elicit a truthful response, to have asked would have been an irrevocable step. What had been obtained from the doctor's own lips could not be easily discounted or refuted. So they played safe, did not enquire and hoped for the best.

> JM: You haven't asked about your prognosis?
> Mrs S: No. I don't want to be told I'm definitely done for. I just put my trust in the doctors and hope that I might get better although I know I might not. There *is* just a chance you know.

I have explained why some patients did not seek to find out about their condition in terms of the relationship between uncertainty and hope. But the converse also requires explanation. Why did other patients seek to establish the truth? How did those who sought to banish uncertainty by seeking to find out about their condition differ from those who did not?

Whether or not patients sought to find out the truth about their condition was, at least partly, a product of their perceptions both of cancer in general and of their own condition in particular. It was not that those patients who sought the truth were not interested in maintaining hope. They most certainly were. It was simply that they believed that they had less chance of losing it completely by asking. They did not regard cancer as being synonymous with death, so, for them, confirmation of the diagnosis did not carry the same degree of threat. They were able to differentiate between various forms of the disease. They recognised that the severity of the illness was variable, that this was partly contingent upon whether it had spread, that it could be contained, and, even, that it could be cured. Those patients who did not see cancer as leading inevitably to death were therefore more likely to seek to establish their diagnosis and to enquire about their prognosis. Having acquired the diagnosis, they would have rid themselves of the uncertainty of not knowing while, at the same time, because they did not make an inevitable association between cancer and death, they could still retain the hope that they would be cured. Their perception of their own condition was also important in this process for, while they did not regard a diagnosis of cancer as necessarily being a death sentence, the converse still held. They were aware that cancer *could* kill. So, in addition to their knowledge that cancer in general could be cured, it was those patients who perceived their *own* condition as being one of the potentially curable ones who were most likely to seek additional information.[5] Whether they enquired or not depended in part, therefore, upon where they located their own condition on their spectrum of curability. For example, there was a noticeable tendency for breast cancer patients to be more likely to enquire about their diagnosis and prognosis. This was possibly partly a result of the publicity given to the condition, especially to the fact that it can be cured. Consequently, those patients may have felt that there was a greater chance of receiving good news. Curiously, patients with melanomas displayed the same tendency. This may have had something to do with the relatively innocuous appearance of the condition and the absence of any other alarming symptoms. On the other hand, those patients who preferred not to know either regarded cancer as being synonymous with death or considered that their own condition was likely to be a relatively serious example of the disease. Consequently, they did not wish, or seek, to have the diagnosis confirmed for, embodied within such a revelation, would have been the inescapable fact that the outlook was poor. Once in possession of the diagnosis they could have held out little hope for the future. 'I don't want to know if it's cancer. I don't want to know I'm doomed.'

So, uncertainty could provide the motivation both for information seeking and for electing to remain in ignorance. Whether or not patients reacted to uncertainty by seeking the truth about their illness depended, at least in part, upon their assessment of the relative likelihood of their receiving good or bad news. This in turn depended upon their conceptions of cancer in general and their own conditions in particular. The only way in which patients with a pessimistic view of the disease could maintain hope was by rejecting, or at least not confirming, the diagnosis. The ways in which patients who did not want to know adjusted to their illness is the subject of chapter 7.

Notes

1. A condensed version of this analysis originally appeared in the *Lancet*. McIntosh, J.; 'Patients' Awareness and Desire For Information About Diagnosed But Undisclosed Malignant Disease.' *Lancet* Vol. II, p. 300, 1976.
2. Kubler-Ross reports a similarly high level of awareness among dying patients (1969, p. 27).
3. It should be pointed out that this type of condition probably constituted a disproportionate number of cases in the particular ward under study.
4. As Davis says, 'uncertainty can be grounds for hope as well as despair' (1966, p. 317).
5. Patients readmitted to the ward for cancer tended to ask fewer questions and to be less desirous of additional information than those admitted for the first time. This was probably because the readmissions had obtained much of the information they wanted during their previous periods in hospital. In addition, though, the fact of their readmission may have alerted them to the possibility that the outlook was not good thereby increasing the risk of receiving an unfavourable response to enquiries about their prognosis and leading to a corresponding reduction in their inclination to ask.

7 PATIENTS WHO DID NOT WANT TO KNOW

Most patients did not react to uncertainty by seeking to find out about the nature and severity of their condition. They preferred the uncertainty consequent upon not knowing because it was precisely this uncertainty which afforded them hope. So long as they did not know for sure, they could always hope for the best. They did not, therefore, attempt to establish the truth about their condition by enquiring of the doctors or in any other way.

But this does not mean that those patients who did not want to know did not seek information or attempt to eradicate uncertainty. They did. However, their information seeking was of a different nature from that undertaken by those who sought the truth. In contrast with the latter, they sought exclusively information which would reinforce their hope. Their response to uncertainty was to attempt to establish and consolidate an optimistic conception of their condition. In their efforts to achieve this, those patients sought, perceived and interpreted selectively those cues which could be taken to indicate either that they did not have cancer or that the outlook was good. The following cases illustrate the ways in which patients who did not want to know attempted to construct and retain hope and avoid realization.

Patients who Suspected their Diagnosis but did not want Confirmation of it or to Receive Information on their Prognosis

This was the largest single category and included 32 patients. While their degree of suspicion could vary, none of them definitely knew that they had cancer. Their desire for additional information was obtained in interviews and supplemented by observation of their interactions with others, particularly that with members of the medical and nursing staff.

Mrs Anderson was a sixty-one year old widow with no family. Her husband had been killed in a road accident seven years previously. I first saw her on the day after her admission to the ward and asked her what she was in for. She replied that she had been admitted for 'breast surgery'.

> JM: What's wrong with the breast?
> Mrs A: I don't know, I never asked. I dressed it myself for two years

then I went to the doctor with my back and blurted it out. But they seem to be very pleased and it doesn't seem to have spread. It must be a sort of cancer but they say it's not under my arm or anything.

JM: Were you told it was cancer?

Mrs A: No. It might be malignant, I don't know. And I don't really want to know either. I'd rather just hope for the best.

JM: How did you know anything was wrong?

Mrs A: Well, I had it for two years and it wouldn't heal.

JM: So you had it for two years—why did you go to the doctor when you did?

Mrs A: Because my back got bad. I thought it might be affecting my back. Until then, I had done everything to keep it from him you know.

JM: Why did you keep it from him?

Mrs A: Well, I'm on my own so I wanted to keep on working. Then when my back got worse I thought I'd had it anyway so I'd better tell him.[1]

JM: What did your doctor say about it?

Mrs A: Well, when I showed him he was just speechless. He was shocked. He probably thought it was worse than it was—but I don't know how bad it is.

JM: Did he say anything else?

Mrs A: He just said that it would have to be treated and that there were no lumps under my arm. He didn't say what it was or anything. And I didn't ask him.

Mrs Anderson was then referred to one of the surgeons who gave her no additional information on the nature of her condition. 'He just said that it wouldn't heal and that it would have to be dealt with. He didn't say exactly what it was. He didn't say it was cancer.'

So, upon admission, Mrs Anderson strongly suspected that she had a malignancy but was comforted by the fact that it did not 'seem to have spread'. However, although not detected until then, axillary node spread was found during her operation. Following her radical mastectomy she was told that there were some 'nasty cells' so they removed her breast and because 'the nodes in the armpit were involved' they 'took them away too'. It was explained to her that she would get radiotherapy 'just to make sure'. I spoke with her again shortly after her operation and asked how she was and what she had had done.

Mrs A: They took off my breast and now I'm going to get radiotherapy treatment.

JM: What is the operation and treatment for?

Mrs A: Well, I don't know. But it wouldn't have healed, they told
me that.

JM: Are you. . .

Mrs A: They didn't tell me about what was inside and what treasures
they found. They did say that the graft was as good as it could
be.

JM: So, are you happy with what you've been told?

Mrs A: Yes. I haven't asked anything. Some people have to know
everything but I don't. I just hope they've got it all—that's all I
hope. I think they have. I hope they have.

Amid all the discouraging signs, such as the fact that the disease had
spread to her armpit and her receiving both an operation and radiotherapy, Mrs Anderson sought reassurance in the observation that this
was the *only* treatment she had received. She interpreted this as meaning that the disease could not have spread any farther.

They haven't done anything else to me—only the breast—so it can't
have spread. So I think I'll probably be OK. If there had been any
more, they'd have found it wouldn't they? That's if it is cancer. It
might not be that at all. I hope not anyway.

So, at that stage, the only change in her orientation towards her illness was a switch from the belief that it had not spread (the nodes had
been 'involved') to the hope that, if it was cancer, the doctors had 'got
it all'. She still did not want confirmation of her suspicion that she had
a malignancy. Her attitude remained unaltered throughout her stay in
hospital. At no time did she ask about her condition, except to enquire
how many treatments of radiotherapy she would receive, and on discharge remained quite content with what she had been told stating that
she did not want to know any more.

JM: Are you happy with what you've been told about your treatment and condition?

Mrs A: Yes. They should tell patients as much as they want to know.
Everything I want to know I've been told. I don't want to know
too much and I think that goes for most of the patients.

JM: So you were able to find out all you wanted to know?

Mrs A: Yes. I think they tell you all you need to know. I don't want
to know everything.

Mrs Anderson was typical of patients in this category. Although she
had a very strong suspicion that she had cancer she did not want confirmation of this and certainly did not want a prognosis. She remained relatively secure in the belief that, if she did have cancer, and she might not,
the doctors had 'got it all'. Above all, she continued to hope.

Mr Laing was admitted with an epithelioma of his tongue. He was a sixty
eight year old retired bus driver with a wife and three married daughters.
He had discovered the growth while eating when, he said, 'I felt it rub-
bing on my teeth'. At first he did nothing about it thinking 'that it would
clear up'. However, when after four months it still had not gone, his
suspicions were aroused and he consulted his GP. 'Because I was afraid
it was something, you know. I'm always afraid of cancer.'
 His brother had died of cancer, which had originated in a carcinoma
of the palate, a few years previously and, since then, the fear of cancer
had always been 'at the back of (his) mind'. So, when admitted to the
ward, Mr Laing had a strong suspicion that he had a malignancy. The
growth had been variously referred to by the doctors as an 'ulcer' or a
'cyst' and he was clearly sceptical of the authenticity of this nomen-
clature. However, at that stage, he felt that it might be better if he did
not know for certain.

JM: What's the trouble?
Mr L: It's a lump on my tongue. They're going to put needles into
 it—radium I think.
JM: What sort of thing is it?
Mr L: It's an ulcer I think. Well, I mean, *they* call it an ulcer. I just
 don't know what it is if it's a cyst or what. I have my doubts
 though.
JM: You still think it could be cancer?
Mr L: Well, it makes you wonder. But they know my brother died of
 cancer and that I was scared stiff of it and maybe don't want to
 tell me.
JM: Would you like to know if it was?
Mr L: Well, I'm not worrying—I'm maybe better not to know.

Mr Laing's suspicions were primarily a product of his lay knowledge
of the disease but they were reinforced by the speed of his admission to

hospital. This he took to be suggestive of his not having a simple cyst or ulcer.

> Mr L: Well, when he said to come in in a week, I really began to wonder you know.
> JM: Wonder what?
> Mr L: If it was something serious.

He regarded the fact that he was to be treated by means of radium as an additional sign that he might have cancer.

> JM: Is there anything you're worried about?
> Mr L: Oh yes, I've worried a lot about my tongue. They've not said what it is. But these needles are not good. They'll be radium needles and they use radium for cancer.

Despite his suspicion, Mr Laing made no attempt to discover whether he had cancer during his stay in the ward. Upon his discharge he still sustained the hope that he might not have the disease and that, even if he did, he would be cured. He had no wish to obtain information which would confound this hope.

> JM: What all have you had done?
> Mr L: I've had seven of these radium needles in my tongue?
> JM: What were they for?
> Mr L: Well, I don't know if it was cancer or what it was. It was a lump in the side of my tongue. It might just be a cyst—I hope that's all it is.
> JM: What made you think it might be cancer?
> Mr L: Well, I just guessed.
> JM: Have you asked if it was cancer?
> Mr L: No, I don't think they would mind though.
> JM: Why did you not ask?
> Mr L: Well, I think I'm maybe better not knowing really.
> JM: What were you told about it?
> Mr L: They didn't tell me anything—just about the needles.
> JM: Would you like to know what it was?
> Mr L: I don't know. I'm not bothered—I'd only worry if I did.
> JM: Are you happy with what you've been told then?
> Mr L: Yes.
> JM: You were able to find out all you wanted to know?

Mr L: Yes—I didn't want to know it all really.

JM: Do you have any worries now?

Mr L: No, not really. Just this thing on my tongue—I just hope it's OK. But I'm not so worried now that I've had the needles. They say it'll be all right. I just hope that's right.

In fact, unfortunately he was not all right. At the end of the study he was readmitted for further treatment.

Mrs Brown was fifty-two and married with one son. She had had a local mastectomy for a malignant breast tumour in the past and when I saw her two years later had been re-admitted with a recurrence in the breast area and lung metastases. She related the history of her condition when I saw her on the afternoon of her admission. She clearly perceived her present condition as a continuation of her previous trouble.

Mrs B: Well, I was in this ward two years ago with a small lump in my right breast which they took out. I don't know if it was malignant or what—I didn't ask.

JM: Was the operation a success?

Mrs B: Well it was up until August this year then it just seemed to fall apart. First I had a stomach bug then I started getting short of breath, which turned out to be fluid on the lung, and then I took bronchitis.

JM: What are you in for now?

Mrs B: I don't know—nobody's told me. My own doctor said there was activity in the blood and I would have the glands at the top of the kidney removed. The activity was activating the wound.

JM: So you went to your own doctor with your symptoms?

Mrs B: Not exactly. I was attending the radiotherapy clinic and I always relied on them. They decided that I would have to come into hospital again. But my own doctor came to see me, he got a letter you see, and told me about the activity in the blood and that there was fluid in the lung.

While she did not challenge the euphemistic description of her condition or seek further information, the explanation offered to her neither informed her of the diagnosis nor did it allay her fears.

JM: Are you at all worried about your condition?

Mrs B: Oh yes, I worried myself into a state of nerves.

JM: What were you worried about?

Mrs B: If I'd ever get better or if I'd anything serious.

JM: What serious thing were you worried about?

Mrs B: Well, if it was cancer or something like that.

JM: Do you think it is?

Mrs B: I just don't know. I haven't asked. I hope not.

JM: You still have the same worry?

Mrs B: Yes, that I won't get better.

JM: Would you like to know if it's a cancer?

Mrs B: No. I think I'd be terribly worried if I knew. I'd rather not.

So, upon admission Mrs Brown was clearly very suspicious and apprehensive but she had not, at that time, sought to determine the exact cause or possible outcome of her illness. She still hoped that she might not have cancer.

At first she had her pleural effusion tapped and then several tests were run 'to help us to decide what to do'. Originally she had been admitted for an adrenalectomy but, on the basis of the results of the investigations and the doctors' deliberations, it was decided that she would be treated by means of drug therapy and that her proposed adrenalectomy would be postponed for the present. This was explained to her.

Now Mrs Brown, we're going to put you on a course of drugs to stop the fluid accumulating in your lung. If the drug works, and we think it will, you won't need to have the operation after all. Once we've seen the chest films we'll see if there's any more fluid to come off and once we've done that we'll start you on the pills. The fluid that's accumulating there is the cause of all your symptoms and if we can stop it accumulating you'll feel much better.

I saw her soon after the above encounter with the doctor and asked if, in view of what he had said, she felt 'any better about things.' Although she remained a very anxious woman, Mrs Brown was heartened by the fact that she would probably not receive the operation. This she took to be an encouraging sign.

Mrs B: A bit. I'm glad I might not get the operation. They probably found it's not as bad's they thought. But I'm still worried—I just hope the drug works.

JM: Did they say what was wrong?

Mrs B: No. They just said that the drug would get rid of the fluid in
    my lung.
JM: Would you like to know exactly. . . ?
Mrs B: Well, I think it's better not to know—you'd only worry if you
    did. She (Mrs Dewar) asks about everything but I'd rather not.

Four weeks later, when about to be discharged, Mrs Brown developed
a chest infection and, because she could have interpreted it as indicating
a worsening of her condition, the doctors felt it necessary to impress
upon her that it was 'just a chest infection' and not another manifestation of her main complaint. 'It's the chest infection that's keeping you
back from getting home. . . It's just a chest infection, it's not the old
trouble coming back.'
    Eventually the infection cleared and she was ready to go home. Her
prognosis was very poor, although there had been some regression of
the disease, but at least her breathing had been eased. She was told
that the drug would continue to work after her discharge and that she
'should be all right now'. At every stage of her treatment, what was
going to be done and, in euphemistic language, why it was being done,
was fully explained to her. She was wholly satisfied with the information
which she had received. The rest, namely the exact diagnosis and the
prognosis, she had no wish to know. When I saw her just before she
went home she was still very anxious about her condition and remained
unconvinced that she was cured.

JM: How are you Mrs Brown?
Mrs B: A bit better. . . but I'm still worried you know.
JM: What about?
Mrs B: That I might not get better.
JM: What makes you think you might not get better?
Mrs B: Well, if it's cancer you see. I don't know if it is.
JM: Have you asked?
Mrs B: No. I haven't asked anything. I leave everything in their hands.
    The less you know is sometimes better. Time enough to worry
    when you hear the worst.
JM: What have you had done?
Mrs B: I had my lung tapped and a course of pills.
JM: Are you happy with your treatment?
Mrs B: Oh yes, they do their very best for you. I'm glad I didn't get
    the operation. That was encouraging.
JM: And you're satisfied with what you've been told about your

condition?

Mrs B: Oh yes. Well, as I said, I'm in good hands and I'm content to let them do what they want because I'd only worry if I knew the details—(laughs) I worry because I don't.

Mrs Brown went home still clinging to the now slender hope that she would be all right. She died shortly afterwards.

Patients who knew the diagnosis but did not want to know their prognosis

The 14 patients in this group all knew that they had cancer on admission to the ward. However, like the previous patients, they had no wish to augment their knowledge once they were there. Specifically, they did not want to know what the outlook for their condition was. Interest in these cases centres upon how they became aware of their diagnosis and their orientations towards their prognosis.

Miss Sheridan, a sixty-six year old retired school teacher, was admitted to the ward with a nodule on her chest at the site of a mastectomy which she had had three years previously. She knew that she had had cancer and that she now had a recurrence of the disease. I asked her what her previous admission had been for.

Miss S: I had a breast removed.

JM: What was wrong with it?

Miss S: A cancerous lump. They never use the word but that's what it was.

JM: What made you think it was cancer if they didn't say?

Miss S: Well I just guessed. It was obvious. They didn't have to tell me. You always think of cancer when you've got a lump and they operated and I got radiotherapy afterwards. And radiotherapy's for cancer. So. . .

JM: Was that operation and treatment a success?

Miss S: Well, I suppose it was up to now but this is me back in with another lump in something the same area.

JM: Sorry, what is it you're in with now?

Miss S: A small lump. It's what they call a secondary. It was a bit of a shock when they found it—I really was upset. But I don't want to put my head in the sand and forget about it. I suppose they'll operate and I'll probably get some X-ray treatment after it. I've had it before. I suppose it's to stop it progressing any further.

The lump had been found during a routine follow-up examination where she was 'just told that they would take me into hospital to see about it'. She was not admitted to the ward until three weeks later and confessed that this had been a period of great anxiety for her. 'That was torture—waiting. You're bound to worry about it. Once you know you want it over as quickly as possible.' However, once admitted to the ward, the operation was performed swiftly and she was informed of its success with a brief, 'Your operation went fine yesterday. Nothing to worry about.' I spoke with her after the operation.

JM: How did it go Miss Sheridan?
Miss S: They said it went well. I just hope that's it now.
JM: Did you ask if it was all right now?
Miss S: No.
JM: Do you intend asking?
Miss S: No. I just hope they got it in time but, of course, you can't tell with cancer. But I'm very glad they got it soon otherwise it would probably just have grown.

After a course of radiotherapy 'to make sure that there are no cells left', Miss Sheridan was ready to go home. She knew that she had been treated for cancer but hoped, because the growth was small and had been attended to promptly, that this might be the end of it. She was aware, however, that she might not be cured and determined not to ask questions pertaining to her prognosis but rather to hope for the best. In any case, she acknowledged that the doctors probably could not give her a definitive answer to such a question.

Miss S: I had a lump removed. It was cancer.
JM: Did they say that?
Miss S: No. But of course I knew.
JM: Are you happy with the treatment?
Miss S: Oh yes. It was small and they got it quickly so I just hope it's all right.
JM: And are you satisfied with what you've been told?
Miss S: Yes. I don't suppose they know the absolute truth. I only hope this is it caught. It could be or it might not. I think they told me what they wanted me to know. But I can understand that with this illness they might not want to tell you too much and worry you.
JM: Do you think there's anything they could tell you that would

worry you?

Miss S: Yes. That I won't get better. I'd rather not know that.

JM: But you wanted to know the diagnosis?

Miss S: Yes. I suppose I really like to know what is wrong. I can meet it better if I know what's wrong rather than wondering.

JM: Are you still worried about it?

Miss S: Well, in my case I worry about progression of it. You just wonder where it might come next if it ever comes back.

JM: But you haven't asked about this?

Miss S: No. I'll just go on hoping. (Crosses her fingers.) But it's always at the back of your mind, 'Is it finished?'.

Mrs Poole, a sixty year old widow was admitted for recurrence of cancer of the breast. She had received treatment for it fifteen months previously and clearly saw her latest admission as being connected with her previous one. She had no doubt, during her first hospitalisation or now, that she had a malignancy. I saw her on the day after her admission.

JM: What are you in for Mrs Poole?

Mrs P: The same trouble as last time—cancer of the breast. Well, it's more or less for the glands underneath my arm—they've something to do with the breast. It's spread from the breast to there or something I suppose. They're going to attend to some glands at the top of my kidneys to control it. I only hope it works.

JM: What treatment did you get last time?

Mrs P: I had radiotherapy treatment.

JM: And did that clear it up?

Mrs P: Well it cleared it up to a certain extent but it just keeps it at bay till the next time. After the treatment I was put on to tablets but I didn't respond very well to the tablets and that's why I'm back in again.

JM: How was it discovered that things were amiss?

Mrs P: I'd been coming for check-ups for a year but things just seemed to get out of control. I'd been coming here regularly every six weeks and Dr Barron said I wasn't responding to treatment and they'd have to take me back in again.

JM: What did you feel about that?

Mrs P: Well, when he explained it to me, that I'd to come in again for more treatment, I just broke down. But I soon came to—I've got to know. I would have been terribly worried if I'd had to go on guessing.

JM: Would you have been more worried?

Mrs P: Oh yes.

JM: Did you ask Dr Barron if it was a cancer?

Mrs P: Well, but I knew that. You just kind of instinctively know I think. And when I saw my own doctor the first time he said, 'You suspect what it might be?' and I said, 'Yes.' There's no point in beating about the bush. I couldn't have stood guessing. I'm one of those people who's got to know.

JM: If you knew that you had cancer what was it that upset you?

Mrs P: The fact that it had got worse and I didn't seem to be getting any better.

JM: So you weren't told it was cancer?

Mrs P: I just knew myself. I would rather know than guessing. If you asked, I think they would tell you if you were really interested. Some would rather not know maybe, but I want to know. They might even ask but not want to know.

JM: How concerned are you about your condition?

Mrs P: I just want to get better and get back to normal.

Mrs Poole knew that she was suffering from a recurrence of a malignancy although she had never been explicitly told that she had cancer. Her awareness was a product of her own knowledge of the disease. This was partly confirmed by her GP's remark that she suspected 'what it might be'. While she maintained that she wanted to know if she had cancer, she acknowledged that some patients might not and, indeed, that even some patients who asked might not 'really' want to know. She was not over-optimistic about her prognosis but hoped that her proposed treatment would work. The treatment was to consist of a combined operation for the removal of her adrenal glands and ovaries in an attempt to check progression of the disease. This decision was imparted to her.

Mr Moorehead: Now Mrs Poole, to clear up your trouble we've decided to remove the glands at the top of your kidneys and your ovaries. They give out hormones which are aggravating your trouble and we find that when we remove them people get much better. But it will mean that you'll have to take a drug, cortisone, for the rest of your life. Now, if you want to know anything else, just ask me.

Mrs Poole: No. Just so long as it helps.

Following her adrenalectomy and oopherectomy she was told that the operation had gone well and that she 'should be all right now.'

JM: How did it go Mrs Poole? What did they do?
Mrs P: They said it went well. I had glands and ovaries removed.
JM: What did they say it was for?
Mrs P: Well, I think I told you before, I had a breast cancer and I had hormone tablets but they weren't suitable for me so they decided to operate instead.
JM: The pills didn't work?
Mrs P: No. They were causing the inflamation to come back again. The operation apparently gets rid of hormones which are causing the trouble to come back. So I hope that clears the trouble up.
JM: Do you feel confident then that you'll be OK now?
Mrs P: Well, they explained that I should be quite all right now—within reason I suppose. I suppose they can't really be certain.
JM: Are you satisfied with the treatment?
Mrs P: Yes. I feel quite satisfied—if I get better.
JM: Will you ask them about the outlook?
Mrs P: No. I know all I think I want to know about it.

Mrs Poole's knowledge of her condition, and attitude towards it, remained unchanged at her departure from the ward. She knew that she had cancer and, while she was aware that her present treatment might not produce a cure, she lived in the hope that she would be all right. She had no wish to threaten tenure of that hope by enquiring further. Accordingly, she did not ask about her prognosis at any time during her hospitalisation. I interviewed her again on the day before she went home.

JM: Your treatment was for cancer you said?
Mrs P: Well, it's really for cancer of the breast. I just hope it helps.
JM: Are you pleased with your progress?
Mrs P: Yes, well if I feel well enough, I feel I'm doing well. I feel fine. So I suppose that's a good sign.
JM: Have you to return to hospital or is this you finished now?
Mrs P: Well, that you never know. I might have to come back in a year's time. I'll have to come back for check-ups anyway.
JM: Are you satisfied with all you've been told?
Mrs P: Yes. Well I think the doctors know best what they're doing without the patient asking too many questions to bother them.

Anyway, there's no point in bothering the staff when I *know*.

JM: What about the outlook for your condition, have you been able to find out enough about that?

Mrs P: (Woefully) Oh, I've known enough. I just hope this will clear up the trouble.

Mr Hutchinson, a gamekeeper, was forty-six and unmarried. He was admitted with a growth in his throat and had no doubt that it was malignant. In fact, apparently his GP had told him that it was 'a sort of cancer'. I saw him during his first day in the ward and asked what he had been admitted for.

Mr H: I've got a growth in my throat. I had a sore throat and a lump came there. I just thought it would go away but when it didn't I thought I'd better see the doctor about it. You worry that it might be cancer, you see, and I got terribly hoarse.

JM: Are you still worried?

Mr H: I don't mind how long it takes as long as I get hope of getting better. It's a sort of cancer you see.

JM: Did they tell you that?

Mr H: Well, my own doctor told me it was a sort of cancer.

JM: Did you ask him?

Mr H: Well, I said, 'I think it's cancer', and he said, 'Well, it's a sort of cancer but they can do a lot for cancer nowadays.' He said he thought it could be cured. I just hope it can.

JM: So you're sure it's cancer?

Mr H: Oh, it's a cancer. There's no doubt about it.

JM: What did the specialist say about it when you saw him?

Mr H: Well, you know what doctors are. They don't tell you much. He didn't say what it was. He just said I'd to come in and get it seen to. He had me in within a week.

JM: What did you think about that?

Mr H: Well, I was a bit anxious at being taken in so quickly. I thought to myself, 'It must be bad if they're in such a hurry.' But I realise that, with the trouble I have, speed is essential. It was a shock certainly.

JM: Are you worried about your condition?

Mr H: Well obviously. It's always at the back of your mind, 'Will it clear up?'

JM: Will you ask about that?

Mr H: No, I'll just take it in my stride and put my faith in the doctors.

So, upon admission, while Mr Hutchinson said that he knew that he had cancer, he found some consolation in the hope that he would be cured. He was not concerned to ask about his prognosis and would be content, as he said, 'as long as I get hope of getting better'. Consistent with this expression of his desire for information, he asked no questions about either his diagnosis or prognosis during his stay in the ward. At first he underwent a number of tests and X-rays designed to detect whether there were any secondary deposits of the disease. Fortunately there were not and he was informed of this. 'The X-rays and tests which we did were all clear. So that's good news.'

It was then decided that his treatment should consist of a course of a new cytotoxic drug, followed by radiotherapy. This decision was conveyed to him, 'We've decided to give you a course of injections with a new drug to dissolve that swelling for you. Then after that we'll give you some radiotherapy to get anything that might be left and to make sure that it won't come back.'

When I spoke with him shortly after this he indicated his delight at the results of the investigations and repeated his hope that the treatment would prove effective.

> Mr H: I'm getting some injections, seemingly something that's quite
>   new. It's a new drug they're trying out.
> JM: Are you a guinea pig then?
> Mr H: I don't mind that as long as it gives me hope of getting better.
>   They've done some X-rays and things, I suppose to find out if it
>   had spread, and they told me that they were clear. So I'm very
>   pleased about that.

He also interpreted the fact that he was not to receive an operation as being an auspicious sign. This, he felt, indicated that his condition was probably not a particularly bad one.

> I'm not getting an operation you see. I don't think my trouble could
> have been bad enough for them to operate on it. They won't operate
> unless they have to you see. So because I'm only getting injections
> and X-rays, I think it's a good omen.

During the course of his treatment the growth shrank and all went well apart from his experiencing considerable discomfort while undergoing the course of radiotherapy. When the treatment was over Mr Hutchinson was told that the growth had 'shrunk considerably' and that he

could go home. He was further informed that the lump would continue
to reduce in size after he was discharged. He left hospital confirmed in
the belief that he had cancer but anxiously clinging to the hope that his
treatment would result in a cure. Although he was aware that this was
not certain he had no desire to obtain information to the contrary.

JM: What have you had done Mr Hutchinson?

Mr H: I've only had injections and the radiotherapy treatment for
the lump in my throat.

JM: What were you told about it?

Mr H: That the injections dissolved the lump and the radiotherapy is
to make sure it won't recur.

JM: Are you satisfied with what you've been told?

Mr H: Yes. The doctors have been very good at keeping me informed.
I've had tests, scans and X-rays and they say they were clear. If I'd
wanted to know any more, I suppose I could have asked. But I
don't think it's all that good to get involved. I don't really want
to know everything.

JM: Is there anything else you'd have liked to have been told about
then?

Mr H: Nothing. Well, you see, I knew I had cancer. And, I mean, you
don't get radiotherapy if it's not cancer and I had radiotherapy to
my throat.

JM: Does that mean you weren't sure you had cancer 'till you got
the radiotherapy?

Mr H: Oh no, I knew all along. That just confirmed it.

JM: So is that you OK now?

Mr H: Well I hope so.

JM: Did you ask about that?

Mr H: No. I just hope I'll be cured. That's my idea so I don't really
want to go boring and asking questions. I think not getting an
operation was a good sign and the tests were clear. I'm just living
in hope. (laughs)

Mr Hutchinson died a year later.

Mrs Baxter's case differs from its predecessors in that she believed that
she knew both her diagnosis and prognosis on admission to the ward.
She was certain that she had cancer and was going to die. However, during the course of her hospitalisation she came to revise her assessment
of her condition and by the time she was discharged had contrived to

convince herself that she did not have the disease after all. In her efforts
to deny her probable fate, she is a striking example of the ways in which
patients attempted to construct hope.

Mrs Baxter was fifty-eight. She arrived in Ward 4C with a fungating
breast mass and axillary involvement. Upon admission she was convinced
that she had cancer and, indeed, it was this belief, together with her perceived hopelessness of her condition, which had, it appeared, played a
significant part in her delay in consulting her doctor. She had made up
her mind that cancer was incurable and that she was going to die. I
asked her what she was in hospital for.

> Mrs B: My breast through neglect. It started eighteen months ago and
>   I never told a living soul. It started as a little lump and it grew
>   and grew and, because I'm a coward, I left it.
> JM: Why were you frightened?
> Mrs B: I just said to myself, 'It's cancer and it's incurable so why
>   bother with the hospital.'
> JM: Why did you go to the doctor in the end?
> Mrs B: Well, when my husband discovered, he got the doctor.
> JM: Had you thought of going yourself?
> Mrs B: No—I was just going to die. I dressed it every day myself.
> JM: How long have you had it?
> Mrs B: A year and a half.

Mrs Baxter did not ask her GP what she had nor did he confirm her
suspicion. She did not need to ask. She felt that she knew. She reported
what transpired when she saw him.

> I told him exactly what I thought and that I was prepared to live
> with it 'till the time came'. He said I was being pessimistic but he
> didn't say it was or it wasn't, he just got in touch with the hospital
> doctors. I also told him that I didn't see about it because I'm a cow-
> ard. He said I couldn't be a coward if I'd lived with that (the belief
> that she was going to die) for eighteen months.

The consultant simply said, 'You know, I think we'll take you in.'
Within a week of seeing him, she was allocated a bed in the ward. Once
in hospital, she said that she felt better now that everything was out in
the open. The strain involved in concealing her condition for so long
had been enormous and she was glad that this was no longer necessary.

I lived that eighteen months on my own all day and had to put a brave face on it when my husband came home at night. But once he knew and my doctor knew, I was a different person. I don't have to hide it anymore and I feel much better now.

At first Mrs Baxter adopted a disturbingly cheerful and open attitude towards her illness and undoubtedly caused other patients some distress. On more than one occasion she was heard to remark, 'It's best to smile. If you go with a smile on your face, St Peter will open the gates more quickly.'

It was decided to operate and it was explained to her that she would receive a radical mastectomy, 'Or else this thing will certainly give you a lot of trouble in the future.' Following her operation she was told, 'Your operation went well. As you see, we removed the whole breast. . . it was just as well that you had it done because there's no doubt that it would have been dangerous if we had left it.'

Subsequent to this her attitude towards her illness changed when a number of cues combined to make her less certain that she had a malignancy. She seized upon this possibility with alacrity and vigour. The first of those cues was the fact that she had had the operation. This she interpreted as being a hopeful sign. On admission she had felt that nothing could be done but having her breast removed gave her a tremendous boost. The fact that something *had* been done suggested to her that perhaps something *could* be done. More importantly though, because she believed that nothing could be done for cancer, it also suggested to her that she might not have that disease after all.

Mrs B: I was surprised that they operated. You see, I didn't think they could do anything. I wish I'd seen about it sooner now. I'd made up my mind that it was cancer, you see, and they say it's incurable, so there was no point in doing anything. But I don't know what it is now.

JM: Do you think it might not be cancer after all?

Mrs B: Well, I don't know. I didn't think they could do anything for cancer.

Shortly afterwards on two separate occasions, she overheard the doctors mention 'ulcers' when deliberating at the foot of her bed. This raised further doubts in her mind about whether she had cancer. Was it possible that she could simply have ulcers? 'When they stand talking at the top of my bed, I listen to what they're saying and two have used the phrase 'ulcers'. Maybe it's ulcers I have, I don't know.'

Having unexpectedly received what she considered to be cause for optimism, Mrs Baxter was not about to readily let go of it. When given the hope that she might not have cancer she sought to confirm it. She therefore immediately set about selectively seeking, and perceiving, cues and pieces of information which would reinforce that interpretation. Any cues which contradicted that conception of her illness, like the fact that her operation was supplemented by a course of injections, were simply discounted. Nor could she risk asking the staff about her diagnosis or prognosis. They might confound her new-found hope.

> JM: Have you asked if it was cancer?
> Mrs B: No. I don't think I want to ask them that now. But I think it mightn't be.

Her reaction was understandable. While most patients who knew that they had cancer were able to maintain some hope for the outlook, because Mrs Baxter associated cancer with death, the only way in which she could construct a hopeful prognosis was by rejecting the diagnosis of cancer. Accordingly, she looked for cues which could be taken to indicate that she did not have the disease after all. She attempted to get clues about her condition both by comparing herself with, and by asking questions of, her fellow patients. More specifically, she sought reassurance from them, and received it. Interestingly she always sought information from patients whom she knew, or thought, to have cancer. 'If I want to know about anything, I go and ask someone I know has cancer about it.'

The other patients did not always take too kindly to this and one remarked to me, 'She's just a pest. She's always talking about her illness. We don't like it.' Nevertheless, they did all appear to feel bound to grant the reassurance which she sought. She quizzed them about the possibility of her simply having ulcers.

> I asked Mrs Beaton and Miss Edwards about it and they said that it could just have been a big ulcer. And lots of other patients seem to think it mightn't be cancer.

Her operation was followed by a course of injections 'just to make sure'. But she did not receive radiotherapy. This did not escape her notice and was to acquire considerable significance in her efforts to construct a hopeful prognosis. She reported having been told by one patient that, 'If they operate and don't give you radiotherapy, that's a good sign.

Although she sounded out her fellow patients on the meaning of her treatment and the possibility of her not having cancer on numerous occasions, I was able to observe only a limited number of these encounters. However, I was present one morning when she approached Mrs Wilson and asked her what she thought was the significance of her not receiving radiotherapy.

> Mrs Baxter: I've heard the doctors talking about ulcers and I'm not getting radiotherapy but other patients are. Does this mean that it's not cancer I've got?
>
> Mrs Wilson: Well, I don't know. It might not be cancer. It might be ulcers.
>
> Mrs Baxter: Well, I think if you don't get radiotherapy it's not cancer. I hope that's right. What do you think?
>
> Mrs Wilson: Well, I've heard you can sometimes get radiotherapy for cancer. I think it's probably a good sign if you're not getting it.

By the time I saw her before she went home, although she was still a little uncertain, Mrs Baxter was relatively hopeful about the outlook.

> Mrs B: They seem to think I'll be all right. They said I could go home and that I shouldn't worry about it. When I came in I was convinced I had cancer. It was silly I suppose. But now I don't think that's what I could have had after all.
>
> JM: Why's that?
>
> Mrs B: Well I heard them talking about ulcers. I hadn't thought that's what it might be. And I didn't get radiotherapy which showed me that I probably didn't have cancer.
>
> JM: So you're sure now that it was ulcers you had?
>
> Mrs B: Well, not one hundred per cent, but pretty sure. I feel so relieved. You see, I thought I was going to die.

Mrs Baxter now had hope where previously she had had none.

Vacillation and Realization

The fact that they were not given their diagnosis or prognosis enabled patients who did not want to know to retain hope and construct an optimistic conception of their condition from the information available to them. Those patients tended to discount, suppress, rationalize or ignore those cues which implied that which they were not prepared to accept. However, such coping mechanisms were not always easy to execute and the perception of certain cues could lead to vacillation of mood and unsolicited realization of the nature and extent of the illness.

Some unfavourable cues, although not sought, could not be easily ignored or discounted and had to be faced. Moreover, even where they could be suppressed or rationalized in some way, they did, nevertheless, have some impact upon the patient. One effect of the impact of such cues was that the patient's mood could fluctuate from day to day or even from hour to hour. This fluctuation in mood was regarded by the ward staff as being particularly characteristic of cancer patients and certainly a considerable number of those in the study evinced this pattern during their hospitalization. Such vacillation between optimism and depression was scarcely surprising since the maintenance of a hopeful fiction was extremely precarious. The patient was constantly being assailed by conflicting signs and evidence and often found it difficult to maintain a hopeful outlook under the impact of a welter of cues to the contrary. His conception of his condition, being in such an unstable state, was therefore likely to vacillate between hope and despair depending upon the weight of evidence supporting either view. This could lead to quite marked and rapid changes in mood.

However, unfavourable cues did not just lead to temporary fluctuations in mood. Some cues, or batteries of cues, were extremely difficult to ignore or explain away and could bring a patient, against his will, to a gradual realization of the severity of his condition. In other words, the weight of evidence was sometimes such that patients were forced to face the truth although they would have preferred not to have known. Certainly, the patient retained hope for as long as possible but for some there came a point when this was no longer possible: the truth had become inescapable. Realization of the true nature and severity of their condition came slowly to those patients through the closing of the alternative interpretations which were open to them. Even then, few patients failed to retain a residue of hope. Patients demonstrated their awareness through the following type of remark:

> I've given up hope now. I don't think they can do any more for me. I think what I have now I'll have for the rest of my days. I don't think they can do much for it.

Often the most potent cue in bringing about this realization was the fact that, despite their expectations and the doctors' assurances, they were not getting any better. Repeated admissions to hospital for treatment was another important indicator.

> This is my third time in here now. I'm not getting any better. In fact I'm getting worse. I think it's only a matter of time now. I don't think they can do anything more for me.

An important attendant question here is how patients reacted to realization. I should point out that a firm realization that the outlook for their condition was hopeless came to only a very small number of patients while they were in hospital. Of those, some adjusted well to this realization and reached a certain acceptance of it while others reacted less well and became very depressed.[2] Unfortunately, the numbers involved are too small to enable us to attempt an explanation of those differing initial reactions. It did appear, though, that those patients who had sought a certain amount of information about their prognosis reacted rather better than those who had not. This, however, remains to be verified.[3]

Having considered how some patients tried to avoid becoming aware, in the following chapter I examine the ways in which others sought to find out about their condition.

Notes

1. In fact, her painful back had nothing to do with her malignancy.
2. Kubler-Ross (1969) has described the ways in which patients come, via a succession of stages, to an ultimate acceptance of the fact that they are dying. At the same time, though, all of them, no matter how much they accepted their terminality, maintained some degree of hope.
3. This question is, of course, outwith the scope of the present study. However, in any research on realization it is probably important to distinguish between patients' initial and ultimate reactions (Shands *et al* 1951). Previous work in the area would suggest that most patients, while perhaps reacting rather adversely at first, ultimately come to terms with the knowledge that they have cancer or that they are dying. (Kubler-Ross 1969, Gerle et al 1960).

8 INFORMATION SEEKING

This chapter examines the ways in which patients who wanted to find out about their condition sought and obtained information. As we have seen, the majority of patients did not desire or seek additional information about their condition preferring instead to maintain as hopeful a conception of their illness as was possible in the circumstances. They had no wish to discover that they had cancer or how serious their condition might be. They preferred uncertainty to knowing the truth. They were therefore perfectly content with the euphemistic accounts of their condition which they received from the medical staff. However, a considerable number of patients responded to uncertainty in a very different way. They sought to eradicate it by finding out the truth about their condition. For those patients the information which the staff volunteered to them was inadequate. They were not fooled or forestalled by what they were told and remained dissatisfied with the euphemistic terms in which the diagnosis was presented to them and sceptical of the prognosis which they were offered. They wanted to know more. How did they set about acquiring additional information? One obvious way of doing so was to enquire of the staff.

Formal Enquiry

Patients who wanted to know knew that they would not be told unless they asked. However, they did not criticise the doctors for not disclosing to them in full without their asking, acknowledging that they had a difficult task to perform and had to be careful not to disclose to everyone. They appreciated that some patients might not want to know and that the doctor therefore had to be guarded in what he said. Thus, they both understood and sympathised with the doctors' tendency to withhold information.

The questions which patients asked about their diagnosis and the sorts of replies which they received were fully explored in earlier chapters. Patients seldom asked explicitly if they had cancer. Much more common were questions like, 'What is it?', 'What's wrong?', and, 'What did you find?' We saw that finding out about one's condition in this way was not easy. In response to those questions, patients would receive a standard euphemistic reply. Most patients did not enquire further: some because they felt this was not likely to prove very profitable and others because they accepted what they were told. Many of the patients believed that the doctors could often be genuinely uncertain of the exact nature of their condition and the prognosis for it and consequently made allowances for the fact that the information which they received in response to enquiry was often less than comprehensive and couched in uncertainty. They believed that they had been told all they could be told. 'I'm sure I've been told all they can tell me. I suppose they can't really be certain. I know with these things they don't know themselves.'

This appreciation of the doctor's uncertainty, which was, of course, to a considerable degree fostered by the doctor himself, probably effectively mitigated what might otherwise have been a hostile indignation at not being told the whole truth. It did, however, also frequently serve to obviate further questioning by the patient.

However, for many patients there was no need to enquire further and, indeed, for some, no need to enquire at all. Not because they believed what they were told to be the whole truth but because they were able to identify what was communicated to them as being euphemistic and to interpret it accordingly. In other words, what they were told contained sufficient information for them to be able to deduce the diagnosis from it. I return to this later in the chapter.

Some patients were not satisfied with the replies which they received and went on to enquire further. Sometimes they would ask the doctor to clarify what he meant: 'What do you mean by activity?' 'What do you mean there are some nasty cells there?' and would receive a relatively more explicit reply but which still stopped short of full disclosure and implied that their condition was only potentially serious: 'It would have gone malignant', or, 'It would have turned into a cancer.' Patients might eventually have to ask directly if they had cancer. The following exchange demonstrates the way in which one patient was gradually forced to become more explicit in his attempt to find out the diagnosis.

Dr Barron: You've got a wart there haven't you?
Mr Symon: What exactly is it doctor?
Dr Barron: It's a little growth but not a dangerous sort of thing.
Mr Symon: Just a growth?
Dr Barron: Well, it's potentially a growth.
Mr Symon: It's not a cancerous thing?
Dr Barron: No. But it might have been if it had been left.

But, even when patients asked outright they were unlikely to receive an unequivocally positive reply. Replies to such direct questions again usually referred to the condition as being potentially serious. 'Well, we don't actually call it a cancer, but, if it had not been removed, it would almost certainly have turned into one. That's why we took it out—to save you having any more trouble with it.' Only if a patient persisted in his demand for the truth was he likely to be told that he had cancer. This disclosure was always balanced by a statement to the effect that the outlook was nevertheless hopeful.

Of those patients who sought information on their prognosis, none wanted to know whether, or when, the illness was likely to prove fatal. They did not want an explicit pronouncement on whether they would live or die. Rather, what they wanted was a progress report or assessment of the extent of the involvement of the disease, that is, how bad their condition was at the present time, or even what its projected course might be, as opposed to whether or not they would survive it. They wanted to know if they were 'clear', if it 'had spread', and whether they would be 'all right now'. That is, they wanted to know whether or not the disease had been vanquished or contained, not whether it was going to kill them.

The extent to which patients wanted to know about the outlook was reflected in the sorts of questions which they asked about it. Enquiry about the prognosis stopped short of asking whether the illness would prove fatal and was restricted to questions concerned with containment and the extent of involvement of the disease: 'Am I clear now?' 'Did you get it all?', 'Has it spread?', 'Will it come back?' and so on. The explanation for patients not asking the ultimate question about their prognosis is again tied up with the maintenance of hope. They wanted to know the truth about their condition, but only up to a point. While they were prepared to accept a setback in their aspirations for recovery, they had no wish to be informed that they were definitely done for, that their case was hopeless. By asking the sorts of questions which they did, they could attempt to find out if the prognosis was good and, at the same time, ensure that the truth, even if unfavourable, would not destroy their hope completely. Given that those patients who asked about their prognosis did not regard cancer as being synonomous with death and were aware that it could sometimes be cured, being told that they were clear of the disease, that it had not spread, or that it would not recur, was taken by them to indicate that the prognosis was good. On the other hand, even an unfavourable reply to their questions would leave some room for hope. Even if they were told that the disease *had* spread or that it had *not* all been removed, they could still maintain the hope that it might be conquered in the future. If they had received an unequivocally positive reply to the question, 'Am I going to die?', no such hope would have been possible.

As outlined previously, the replies which patients received to questions about their prognosis were optimistic ones. The doctors' main concern was to ensure that they left them with hope for the outlook, whether such hope was entirely justified or not. It was therefore not at all easy for patients to obtain a frank assessment of their prognosis. They would not be told that the disease had not been entirely eradicated or that there was a possibility that it would recur. Even in cases where the doctor knew the outlook to be grim, the patient would be given to believe that everything was under control.

No patient asked, 'Am I going to die?' or, 'How long have I got to live?' Probably the nearest patients got to this was by asking if they would be 'cured'. Only two patients did so. They received reassuring replies.

> Dr Ogston: Well Mr Urquhart, you'll be getting home next week.
> Mr Urquhart: Will I be cured then?
> Dr Ogston: We hope so. We're not giving you these injections for
> fun. (laughs).

Mr Urquhart did not survive his lung cancer.

We can see, then, that patients who asked questions about their condition did not always receive as candid a reply as they would have wished. Instead they were replied to in accordance with routine responses which assumed that they did not want to know. Given that the doctors were unable to discriminate accurately between those patients who genuinely wanted to know and those who did not, this was the only way in which they could manage their uncertainty. All this does not mean that patients were unable to find out anything by asking, simply that it was difficult for them to do so and that they often obtained less information than they sought. A major barrier to their efforts to find out about their condition was the fact that the doctors were clearly uncertain about the status of patients questioning: did they really want to know and, if so, how much did they want to know? In other words, what constitutes asking?

What Constitutes Asking?

This question is clearly central to any discussion of whether, and how much, patients want to know about their condition. To what extent is

their desire for information reflected in what they ask? The short answer
is that the patients wanted to know precisely what they asked: if they
asked what they had, they wanted to know what they had, and if they
asked if they were 'clear', they wanted to know exactly that, no more
and no less. In other words, when they asked about their diagnosis and
prognosis they wanted a straight answer. Certainly all those who asked
would have liked to have been told that they did not have cancer or
that the outlook was good but this does not mean that they did not
want the truth. What they would have preferred and, indeed, what
they probably hoped for, and what they wanted to know, were very
different. They hoped for a favourable assessment but wanted to be
told the truth even if it was bad news. The fact that all those who asked about their condition during this study wanted a frank response is
especially important in view of the staffs' belief that many patients who
asked simply wanted reassurance. Those patients who did not want to
know did not dare to ask. To have sought reassurance in this way would
have been to have risked finding out that they had cancer or that the
outlook was poor. After all, *they* did not know that the doctors would
regard their questions as requests for reassurance and not as being
indicative of a desire for the truth. As far as the patient was aware the
doctor would give him a frank reply. So, it was only those patients who
genuinely wanted to know who asked questions about their condition.

Having said all that, it must be conceded that, while all the patients
in this study who asked about their diagnosis in relatively inexplicit
ways: 'What is it?' 'What did you find?' did want to know if they had
cancer, there is always the chance that patients could ask that sort of
question in innocence of the sort of reply which it could elicit and
might be shocked to be told, 'It's cancer.' It might, therefore, be un-
wise to disclose to patients who ask about their diagnosis in this relatively inexplicit way. In any case, in the present study most patients who
were dissatisfied with the replies which they received to their initial
questions would go on to ask the more explicit questions: 'Is it cancer?'
and 'Is it malignant?' For others, of course, the euphemistic reply was
itself sufficient to confirm their suspicions. Every patient who asked
if he had cancer or a malignancy wanted to know. They had not reached
the decision to ask this question lightly and were both aware of the possibility that they had the disease and prepared to accept it. Given the
unequivocal and irrevocable nature of these questions, this probably
applies to all patients who ask them.[1] So, while one cannot assume
that patients who ask in relatively inexplicit ways want to know
(although the present study suggests that they probably do), it is likely

that all those who ask explicitly if they have the disease want to know the truth.

While patients who asked about their prognosis wanted some assessment of the outlook, they did not want to be told that they were going to die. They simply sought a truthful response to the sorts of questions which they asked. Among the questions which patients asked relating to the outlook was: 'Will I be all right now?' Care is required in its interpretation. It is similar in nature to questions like: 'What is it?' insofar as it does not contain any indication that the patient suspects cancer and is the sort of question which might be asked routinely by any hospital patient. Other questions relating to the prognosis could not. Questions such as: 'Did you get it all?', 'Has it spread?' and 'Am I clear now?' are clearly associated with an awareness of at least the possibility of having cancer. They refer to specific features of malignancy such as spread, recurrence and difficulty of eradication and are therefore likely to be specific to that disease. As such, they are not the sort of question which any hospital patient might ask. They are only likely to be asked by patients who are aware that they have, or might have, cancer and constitute a specific attempt to elicit information on the prognosis for that disease. All the patients in this study who asked that sort of question wanted a limited, but truthful, assessment of their prognosis. Limited in the sense that they did not want to be told if they were going to die and truthful in the sense that they were prepared to accept that they might not yet be cured or that the disease had not yet been completely eradicated.

Finally, some patients may hope to obtain information pertinent to the nature and progress of their condition by asking questions about their treatment and tests: 'What are these pills for?', 'How were the X-rays?', 'Were the tests OK?' and so on. This device was certainly used by some of the patients in the study who wished to find out about their condition but it can never be assumed that such questions are always, or even usually, a request for a frank rendering of the diagnosis or prognosis.

Whom did they Ask?

When patients wanted to find out about their diagnosis or prognosis they would nearly always ask a doctor. By and large, the nursing staff were not regarded as an appropriate source for this sort of information. This is not, of course, to say that they were never asked those sorts of questions. Some patients would enquire of anyone: 'If I felt they could tell me, I would ask anybody.' It was simply not nearly so frequent an

occurence as one might imagine. What this meant was that, contrary to
expectations, the nursing staff were not bedevilled by awkward questions from patients about the nature of their condition. The main reason
for patients not asking them was their belief that they did not possess
the information which they sought.

> I never asked questions of the nurses because I knew they weren't in
> a position to tell me. They weren't informed. They wouldn't know.
> It's not their job.

> I'd go straight to the top, to a doctor, and ask. I wouldn't ask any-
> one but a doctor. They would know more about it than a Sister or
> a nurse. The nurses wouldn't know much about it.

Many patients also appreciated the fact that, even if they did know,
the nurses were probably not allowed to disclose certain types of
information to them and that, in consequence, it would be unfair to
question them about certain matters.

> They're not allowed to tell and it might cause trouble for them if
> they said something they shouldn't say.

> I wouldn't ask the nurses. It's putting too much of an onus on them.
> They might say something they'd get into trouble about later.

Those patients who did question the nursing staff tended to restrict
their queries to the Sister or senior nurses.

That the patients' reluctance to question the nurses about their condition was not due to diffidence, or because they found them unapproach-
able, is demonstrated by the fact that they did not hesitate to ask them
about a whole number of other things. Indeed, when it came to other
enquiries they were far more likely to ask the nurses. The information
which patients did seek from them tended to be of a more general nature: how their wound was doing, whether the stitches were OK, when
they had to go for treatment, and about the rules on visiting and telephone use and so on. Their reluctance to seek information from the
nursing staff was therefore confined solely to questions relating to their
diagnosis and prognosis.

While the patients had reservations about questioning the nurses, all
the doctors were regarded as fair game when it came to finding out
about their condition. Many patients saw the medical staff as a team

and would enquire of any of them. However, not even all the doctors
were regarded by all patients as being equally appropriate sources of
information. A substantial number of them preferred to approach particular members of the medical staff. The most popular choice by patients was the consultant in charge of their case. He, they felt, would
be best able to answer their questions. 'I asked Mr Donald. Well, he did
the operation and knows more about my history than any of the others.'

For other patients the opportunities available for questioning particular doctors, their personal liking for them, and how at ease they
felt with them, were important considerations governing whom they
asked. This tended to bias those patients towards the junior doctors
with whom they had more contact and whom they regarded as being
more approachable.

Dr Dunlop. He's round every day and he's easy to get on with.

I'd ask Dr Ogston or Dr Samuel. These are the two I've been most
used to. Dr Samuel has a very nice manner.

Dr Craib because I like him.

However, we have already seen that whoever patients asked they were
likely to find it extremely difficult to find out what they wanted to
know. In view of this, it was possible that they would resort to certain
tactics to obtain the information which they sought.

Patient Tactics

The most notable thing about patient tactics was the relative absence of
them. The great majority of patients who sought information did so by
asking directly and with a complete lack of guile. Persistence was
usually the only weapon which they employed. Apart from the patient
who I am convinced pretended to be asleep in order to overhear what
the doctors would say about him when they arrived at his bedside—he
certainly 'awoke' abruptly, when they left—only a handful of patients
resorted to alternative strategies for getting information. The most common of those was for patients to ask the same question of different
doctors to see if their replies matched. This tactic had, of course, little
chance of success as the routinized nature of the doctors' responses
ensured consistency in what the patient was told by different members
of staff. Asking questions about their treatment may have been another
roundabout way in which patients hoped to get information about their

condition. If such was the case, clearly, as we saw earlier, such questions did not achieve the desired result.

No patient invoked his 'right' to be told about his condition and apart from one woman, who used the refusal of injections as a bargaining counter in order to find out about her condition, no other patient refused treatment, threatened to discharge himself from hospital or appeared to engage in any other form of bargaining for information. However, while patients did not employ subterfuge in order to obtain information, there were other indirect ways in which they were able to find out about their condition. One of those was through the perception and interpretation of cues.

Cues and Symbols

For patients who wanted to find out about their condition much information was available to them informally in the shape of cues and symbols which indicated the nature and extent of their illness. Of course the interpretation of those cues required the patients to have at least a suspicion that they had cancer. Had they not suspected, the cues would not have had the same significance for them.

There were three main ways in which patients were able to obtain confirmation of their diagnosis without being explicitly told.

Firstly, the treatment which they received was a powerful clue for many of them. The fact that they had had an operation was often taken as confirmation that they must have had a malignancy.

JM: Were you told it was cancer?
Mr B: They didn't need to. I knew when they did the operation that it must have been cancer.

Similarly, the receipt of radiotherapy was regarded by many as a strong indicator that they had cancer. 'Well, you see, I knew I had cancer. I mean, you don't get radiotherapy if it's not cancer and I had radiotherapy to my throat.'

Secondly, the fact that they were not informed of their diagnosis by means of an explicit and recognizable label helped to confirm for some patients that they had a malignancy. It was assumed that an unthreatening diagnosis would be disclosed to them and the absence of such a disclosure was taken to indicate that their condition must be something more sinister. This was reinforced by the commonly held belief that the doctors would not tell them that they had cancer.

Thirdly, many patients deduced the diagnosis from what the doctors told them. The important point here is that the patients interpreted what they were told in accordance with the conception of their condition which they wished to maintain. So, in the case of patients who wanted to know the diagnosis, with their suspicions providing the interpretative framework, the euphemisms employed by the doctors were often seen for what they were and interpreted accordingly. Thus, 'suspicious cells', 'nasty cells', and so on were often taken to mean cancer. Although, occasionally, a patient would ask the doctor to clarify what he meant, 'What do you mean there's some activity there?', usually, the patient who wanted to know knew that they were euphemisms. In other words, the diagnosis was implicit in the doctors' statements for many who wished to obtain it. On the other hand, for those patients who did not want to have their suspicions confirmed, what they were told was sufficiently ambiguous to allow them to maintain the conception that they might not have cancer and to retain their hope. For them, 'suspicious cells' could be interpreted as meaning that the diagnosis was equivocal and that they might not have cancer after all. Taken together, these ways of finding out meant that many patients obtained confirmation of their diagnosis without having to ask for it directly and without being explicitly told.

The fact that many patients were able to deduce what they had from what they were told raises the question of what constitutes telling. The patients were not explicitly told what they had and could not, therefore, be said to have had the information formally conveyed to them. What they were told merely embodied certain clues about their condition. Communication of the 'truth' depended upon the interpretation of those clues. However, the fact that patients were often able to interpret such cues correctly means that the doctors clearly 'told' them much more frequently than they imagined. This was not, of course, their intention nor were they aware that they had done so. What happened was that the suspicious patient who wanted to know the truth was able to interpret what he was told in accordance with these suspicions. He was able to tune into the doctor's wavelength when he talked about his condition in terms of 'activity', 'suspicious cells' and so on and to know precisely what he meant. In such cases the doctor was telling without being explicit and without intending to do so. At the same time, this euphemistic form of communication enabled those patients who did not wish to have their diagnosis confirmed to retain the belief that they might not have cancer. They could conclude that the vagueness of the stated diagnosis simply reflected the equivocal nature of their condition or, alternatively, such clues could simply be discounted. In those cases, clearly the doctor was not telling. The essence of telling in this context therefore lay not in what was communicated to patients but in the patient's own attitude towards discovering the truth about his diagnosis and his consequent interpretation of what he was told. It is revealing that patients very seldom questioned the euphemisms used by the doctors. They either understood what they meant or had no wish to have their meaning elaborated upon.

That patients were able to deduce their diagnosis from what they were told is not so very surprising when we consider that the fact that the doctors employed euphemisms, in itself, meant that their communication to patients was bound to contain some clue as to the nature of their condition. Euphemisms like, 'nasty cells', 'suspicious cells', 'activity', 'might become dangerous', 'it hasn't spread' or 'it's clear' all make oblique reference to the truth: that the patient has a malignant condition. Nor could it be otherwise. Euphemisms by their very nature must contain some relevance to the subject to which they refer. In this case they alluded to certain distinctive characteristics of cancer. Had they not done so, they would not have been euphemisms: they would have been lies.

The implications of the above discussion are clear. In many cases, the doctors effectively communicated their diagnosis to patients who wanted to know without mentioning cancer or malignancy. Whether the doctor 'told' or not depended upon the patient's desire to know the truth. The patients whom he told in this way were self-selective in that only those who wanted to know would interpret what they were told as meaning that they had cancer.

Patients also sought information on the outlook for their condition through the interpretation of cues. However, the quest for information from informal sources was by no means confined to those patients who wanted to find out the truth about their prognosis. On the contrary, the great majority of patients who did not want to know also made use of this source. Both categories of patient did so in order to reduce uncertainty, not by finding out the truth, but by constructing a hopeful prognosis out of the variety of cues available to them. Attempting to eliminate uncertainty by seeking to find out the truth was the exception rather than the rule. The majority of patients sought information which would reinforce their hope. The two groups perceived different cues and interpreted the same ones differently in accordance with whichever kind of certainty they wished to establish. Those patients who were only interested in a hopeful interpretation of their prognosis sought, perceived and interpreted selectively those cues which could be taken to indicate that the outlook was good. In their efforts to establish this kind of certainty, the information seeking engaged in by those patients was highly selective in that only information which would allow the construction and tenure of an optimistic prognosis was entertained. Any evidence to the contrary was simply ignored or suppressed.

An obvious question here is, why did those patients who wanted accurate information on their prognosis make use of informal sources at all? Why did they not simply ask for the information which they desired and leave it at that? Was it as hypothesized, and, that restriction of formal communication to the patients and lack of success in information seeking within the formal channels led them to seek information within the informal context? Well, certainly some patients turned to informal sources for this reason but most of those who enquired intimated that they were satisfied that, in response to their enquiries, they had been told as much as they wanted to know. For example, if they asked if they were 'clear' they would be told if they were. Why, then, did they also use the interpretation of cues and symbols as an information resource?

One reason was that they did not quite know whether to trust what the doctors told them. While the doctors would presumably tell them if they were clear of the disease, would they also tell them if this were not the case? The patients were aware that the doctors might wish to conceal certain facts from them in order to spare them anxiety: 'He might just be saying that so as not to worry me.' However, they had no way of knowing when they might be doing so. In other words, they had no way of telling whether what they were told was the truth or whether the doctor was merely offering reassurance. Such formal information therefore had to be checked. The patients could only check whether what they were told was a reliable indication of how they were progressing by observing what happened to them. Informal information seeking was therefore employed both to check and supplement what they had been told. Thus, even when they received reassuring replies, those patients would continue to scrutinise the cues which they encountered in an effort to modify or augment their formally obtained knowledge about the prognosis. It was not that their questions had been left unanswered or that they *knew* that information was being withheld from them, but rather a feeling that the doctors *might* not be presenting them with the whole picture which led them to do this. Nor was this simply an idle attempt to confirm the reassurances which they had received. They sought the truth and were prepared to face it. With those patients, formal and informal information seeking would often be carried out simultaneously.

Part of the explanation for those patients making use of informal sources is even more simple than that. Patients who want to find out about certain things are not likely to ignore the evidence of their own senses. It would, therefore, have been surprising if the patients who wanted to find out about their prognosis had *not* made use of informal sources. The endeavour involved little effort other than observing and interpreting what was happening to them. It was therefore, almost inevitable that such information, being freely available, should be incorporated into their conceptions of the outlook.

Not all patients who sought information on the outlook in this way also sought information formally. Those patients could not, therefore, be said to have been diverted to informal sources by a failure to obtain what they wanted to know from the staff. Nor were they discouraged from asking by an anticipation that they might not be told the truth. On the contrary, they feared that if they asked they might be told more than they wanted to know. Remember, those patients who sought to find out about their prognosis only wanted to know about it up to a point. They did not want to find out that they were going to die and, in enquiring directly, there was a risk of being told precisely that. Accordingly, those patients who were not prepared to take that risk concentrated exclusively upon trying to find out what they wanted to know from informal sources. The patient had a far greater measure of control both over the information obtained within the informal context and over the meaning which he derived from it. Because informal information was amenable to selective perception and different interpretations, the pursuance of information from this source carried far less risk of obtaining the sort of unequivocally grim information which the patients did not desire. If information from that quarter suggested that which patients were not prepared to accept, it could be more easily discounted. The patient could, therefore, to a considerable extent, discover as much or as little as he wanted to know. It was for this reason that some patients who wanted to find out about their prognosis used the interpretation of cues and symbols as their sole source of information.

This element of control was also, of course, central to the choice of this source of information by those patients who sought only to construct an optimistic assessment of their prognosis. They too could make use of the malleability of such information. They could select those items which could be taken to indicate a hopeful outlook and ignore or discount those pieces of information which did not comply with what they wanted to believe or which could not be interpreted favourably. Thus, the attraction of the informal context for many patients was that information obtained therein, if perceived selectively and interpreted appropriately, could be used either to support a favourable conception of the outlook or to ascertain as much of the truth as the patient was prepared to accept. Information obtained formally would have been much less subject to such processes.

The cues available to patients were many and varied. They differed considerably in the weight and significance which they carried and the degree to which they were amenable to alternative interpretations. Some cues were much less pliable than others and some inauspicious ones could only be managed by their suppression. Moreover, the significance of particular cues also varied from one patient to another. For example, the fact that a patient died from what originated as a cancer of the breast might not have been of great significance for a patient with a growth in her mouth but it certainly could be for another patient with breast cancer. Just as cues had different degrees of salience for different patients, different patients also interpreted the same cues differently. With patients who sought the truth their interpretation was dependent upon their conception and knowledge of the disease and its treatment. Some patients, for instance, regarded the fact that they were treated by means of radiotherapy as an indication that their prognosis was bad while others interpreted it as a good sign. This, in turn, depended upon the meaning which they ascribed to radiotherapy. However, the meaning which patients who sought only an optimistic interpretation of their condition derived from cues was not just a product of preconceptions about the nature and treatment of cancer. Those patients interpreted cues in accordance with the particular conception of their condition which they wished to construct. This could lead to radical modification of their interpretative frameworks. Preconceptions about the meaning of particular cues would often be changed in accordance with what the patient wanted them to suggest. Previous beliefs about the significance of a particular cue could be abandoned, the patient constructing from it the interpretation which most accorded with whatever conception of his condition he wished to hold. If cues *could* be interpreted hopefully, they were seized upon with alacrity as constituting further proof that the outlook was good. If not, they would be suppressed.

What cues did the patients use in the construction of their prognosis and how did they interpret them? The main cues were associated with the sort of treatment which the patients received. However, even before they received any treatment at all, the time which the medical staff took to reach a decision on the appropriate form of treatment was regarded by some patients as an indication of the severity of their condition.

Some patients felt that delay in reaching a decision and instigating treatment probably meant that their case could not be very urgent while others interpreted what they perceived as being a delay as meaning the opposite. They feared that the reason the doctors were taking a long time to come to a decision was because their condition might be serious and complicated. 'I just wonder why they're taking so long to make up their minds about what they're going to do. I hope it doesn't mean that it's a very serious thing I've got and they're not sure how to tackle it.'

Irrespective of the time taken to reach decisions, patients certainly appeared to be less anxious after their operation, or the beginning of treatment, than they were prior to it. In part this reflected their relief that action had been taken at last and that their operation was now behind them[2] but, in addition, some patients regarded the fact that they received an operation or treatment at all as being a hopeful sign: because something *was* being done it suggested that something *could* be done and that their case therefore was not hopeless. 'I was bothered about it before the operation but after I had it done I didn't think so much about it. I didn't think there was anything they could do you see.'

The type of operation which a patient received often acted as a clue to the severity of their condition. Patients distinguished between 'big' and 'small' operations. For example, a radical mastectomy was taken to indicate a more advanced condition than that which only required removal of the breast. A second operation was invariably regarded as a sign that the condition was fairly well advanced. Some patients did not receive an operation at all and interpreted this as being a good sign. Being treated by means of radiotherapy instead was often taken to indicate that their condition was not serious enough to warrant surgery.

> Oh Yes. And I'm glad I didn't get an operation like some of the other patients. That's probably because mine is surface and not deep down like their's. I got a course of drugs followed by radiotherapy and the lump has certainly shrunk.

> I only had radiotherapy. I didn't get an operation. I suppose it's because I'm not as bad as some of the others.

However, other patients ascribed a different meaning to receiving radiotherapy instead of an operation. They interpreted this as an indication that their condition was worse than those who were operated upon. 'I'd rather have had an operation. It's not good when they just give you X-ray treatment. It means you're worse than them that get operations.'

Many patients, of course, received both an operation and radiotherapy. Whether or not their operation was supplemented by this form of treatment was perceived by many of them as being an important indicator of how bad their condition was. Such additional treatment was usually regarded as a bad sign and, consequently, the news that they were not to get it was received with considerable relief.

I got some good news this morning. I'm not getting radiotherapy after all. That really gave me a lift. It showed me it isn't as serious as I thought.

An aunt of mine had a breast removed and is very well. But she didn't have radiotherapy after her operation so I suppose mine must be worse.

While it was a useful cue for those patients who wanted to enhance their knowledge about the severity and possible outlook for their condition, patients did not inevitably interpret the addition of radiotherapy as a bad sign. Those patients who sought only an optimistic assessment of their prognosis were able to interpret the fact that they got radiotherapy differently or to revise their understanding of what it meant to receive it. They rationalized its addition in the same terms in which the doctors explained its use to them: 'It's just a safeguard'; 'They're just making sure'; 'This ensures that there'll be no more trouble'. By those means, those patients who were not prepared to accept indications that the outlook might be bad contrived to explain the fact that they received radiotherapy in a relatively unthreatening way.

The receipt of other forms of treatment was subject to the same variety of interpretations as radiotherapy. The only difference was that they were not so readily associated with the treatment of malignancy and were, therefore, more amenable to optimistic interpretation. This was particularly so when they were the only form of treatment employed. Thus, to receive drugs instead of an operation was more likely to be interpreted as a good sign than receiving radiotherapy on its own. However, if such treatment was used to supplement an operation, then, like the addition of radiotherapy, it was often taken to be a bad indication. 'They say I'm all clear then they give me more treatment. I just don't understand it. Maybe I'm not clear after all. . . I'm worried sick about it.'

Other patients were able to rationalize the fact that they received supplementary treatment. 'Well, the injections are just to make sure that everything will be all right.'

The tests which they underwent, depending upon when they were carried out, provided a further potential set of cues for patients. Tests carried out prior to treatment were usually perceived as being normal and routine. After all, the doctors had to find out about the nature of their problem. But investigations *after* the operation or treatment were a different matter. Such investigations could mean that the doctors were not convinced that the disease had been entirely eradicated. Were they looking for evidence of spread? Had it spread? How far advanced was it? The results of these tests were anxiously awaited. Negative findings were very reassuring. They had been investigated and were pronounced clear. On the other hand, if additional treatment was implemented on the basis of the investigations, this provided a clear sign to many patients that the disease had spread or, at least, had not been eradicated.

As one would expect, patients also sought to acquire information by trying to overhear what the doctors said to each other about their cases: 'They would talk among themselves and you had to try to glean from that.' However, the staff's communication was so guarded that this was not a very profitable exercise. Very little information could be obtained in this way. Moreover, the interpretations put upon extracts from such discussions could be mistaken. As we saw, for example, Mrs Baxter, upon overhearing a discussion of her case, came to believe that she could simply be suffering from ulcers.

If attempting to glean information from the doctors' deliberations was not a very fruitful pursuit, what they did *not* say was sometimes regarded as being of great significance. While patients did not expect their diagnosis to be volunteered to them, not being given an explicit diagnosis in response to enquiry could be interpreted as being a bad sign. In other words, if the doctor seemed to be withholding information, some patients took it to mean that their condition was probably serious. Other patients were able to manage and rationalize not being given an explicit diagnosis by ascribing uncertainty to the doctors: their replies were ambiguous because they could not be sure. For them, therefore, such euphemistic responses could be regarded as a hopeful sign.

Another, and continuing, source of information for patients was their perception of their own physical progress: whether they felt any better, whether their growth had diminished in size and so on. Such things were felt to be important barometers of how well they were doing and, hence, of the possible outlook.

> Yes, well if I feel well enough I feel I'm doing well. I feel fine. So I suppose that a good sign.

Whenever I saw the swelling go down I knew it was OK.

Signs of improvement in their condition were sought assiduously and, in this state, even to be told that they were looking better served to boost their hopes. Some of those who saw little improvement in their condition were able to comfort themselves with the thought that it would 'take time'.

Clearly, cues formed an important part of the patients' information network. However, this was also something of which the ward staff were well aware. Consequently, they attempted to exercise some measure of control over the cues available to them.

Management of Cues

Clearly, not all information obtainable from informal sources could be controlled by the staff. They knew this and simply tried to restrict its volume as far as possible. While much of the management simply entailed taking care to avoid transmitting certain cues to patients, some of it involved deliberate manipulation in order to counteract specific cues by either influencing the patient's interpretation of them or by reducing their incidence.

In their efforts to avoid transmitting cues, the doctors had to be careful in what they did. Take the case of a woman who developed bruising on her back. It was first spotted by the sister who asked the resident if he would have a look at it. As he prepared to attend to the matter at once, she cautioned him.

No, not just now. Do it casually when you're looking at something else because she is very anxious and worries about every little thing.

In this way, she hoped to avoid drawing attention to something which the patient could interpret as meaning that something further was wrong.

They had, of course also to be very careful in what they said. All communication to patients was geared to avoiding the transmission of cues to them and to counteract the influence of other potentially unfavourable ones. This was mainly achieved by presenting as hopeful a picture of their condition as possible. For example, a patient whose case was acknowledged to be hopeless might be told that some time had been spent in deciding what form of treatment he would receive after discharge in order to lead him to believe that his condition was worthy of extensive deliberation and therefore, by implication, was still eminently treatable.[3] These optimistic presentations were fully explored in chapters 3 and 4. But in addition to this more general effort to manage awareness and instill optimism, the doctors would also attempt to counteract the influence of specific cues by what they told patients. For example, being aware that patients might put pessimistic interpretations upon the receipt of tests, the doctors presented them to them as being a matter of routine. In this way, they endeavoured to render them non-threatening. Similarly, additional treatment was explained in terms of 'making sure'. They would also attempt to neutralise the potential cue of a patient being admitted to hospital very quickly: 'It just happens that we have a spare bed at the moment.'

In addition to *what* they communicated, the *way* in which they did so was also regarded as being important in managing patient's interpretations. The doctors therefore avoided treating the patient's condition with too great solemnity. Humour might be employed to reinforce this attempt to persuade the patient that his condition could not be too bad.

More deliberate manipulation was effected in relation to the reputation of the ward and its staff. The doctors knew that Ward 4C was fairly widely known as 'the cancer ward' and that its medical staff were also, to some extent, recognised as cancer specialists. This they did their best to contain. To be known as the cancer ward was bad enough, but to acquire a reputation as a death ward would have been much worse. The medical staff attempted to avoid the growth of such a reputation by avoiding death on the ward as much as possible. This was achieved by transferring terminal patients, where practicable, to one of the smaller peripheral hospitals.[4] But this had to be carefully managed in case the patient took his transfer to mean that they were giving up on him. There was little the doctors could do to influence their personal reputation as cancer specialists but attempted to do so on the few occasions when they could. For example, one of the surgeons gave a public lecture on cancer. On learning afterwards that the press had been present, he made a point of contacting the newspaper to ask them not to print his name in case it led people to associate him with cancer.

Another attempt at manipulation was seen in the use of treatment in the management of cues. The doctors were careful to avoid letting a cessation of treatment indicate to a patient that his condition was hopeless or that they had abandoned his case. They might, therefore, continue to treat a patient even when they believed that it would probably do no good. Similarly, the doctors might occasionally give the patient some form of treatment, usually drugs, partly in order to make them feel that something was, and therefore could, be done.[5] I must emphasize, though, that patients were not given treatment or operated upon simply in order to help allay their anxieties. Only if there was uncertainty about whether to proceed with a particular form of treatment could this consideration tip the balance. Nevertheless, it was a factor which carried some weight in such marginal decisions.

Finally, the staff were also aware that the patients might obtain information by conversing, or comparing themselves, with other patients with the same or a similar condition. In an attempt to get round this, they avoided placing such patients next to one another on the ward. This worked so long as the patients were confined to bed but if they were ambulant, and it only required one party to be so, like very soon sought out like. As this would indicate, informal information seeking did not just consist of the interpretation of cues. Other people with whom the patients came into contact while in hospital, for instance relatives, fellow patients and other hospital personnel, were also a potential source of information. Those parties constitute the informal network. It is examined in chapter 10. The next chapter documents some of the careers of patients who wanted to know about their condition.

Notes

1. Unfortunately, and possibly surprisingly, questions like, 'I don't have cancer do I?' or, 'It's not malignant is it?', which are customarily interpreted as being requests for reassurance that patients do not have the disease, were not posed during the course of the study. I cannot, therefore, say anything about the sort of response which patients hoped to obtain to these questions. However, their hesitant quality would suggest that the patients who ask these questions are indeed seeking reassurance.
2. One patient observed, '. . . waiting for something to be done. Once the treatment starts the anxiety eases. I think it's fear of the unknown.'
3. Glaser and Strauss have described the 'situation as normal' tactics employed by staff in interaction with dying patients. 'Awareness Contexts and Social Interaction'. *American Sociological Review,* Vol. 29, No. 5, 1964, pp. 669-78, p. 672.
4. By no means all such patients could be transferred. Moreover, the majority of patients were, of course, transferred simply for convalescence or to finish off their course of treatment.
5. This tendency to 'do something' in order to manage patients' awareness has also been noted by Glaser and Strauss (1965, p. 186).

9 PATIENTS WHO WANTED TO KNOW

This chapter is devoted entirely to presenting some typical careers of patients who wanted to find out about their condition. The extent of their desire for information varied: some only sought to know their diagnosis while others wanted to find out about the outlook for their condition as well. Those patients wanted to know the truth and in an attempt to obtain it sought information from both formal and informal sources.

Patients who Suspected their Diagnosis, wanted Confirmation of it, but did not want their Prognosis

This category was composed of nine patients who suspected that they had cancer and who desired, and set out to obtain, their diagnosis. They did not, however, want an accurate assessment of their prognosis. While they were prepared to accept that they had cancer, these patients preferred to retain hope for the outlook rather than seek to find out about it.

Mrs Craig was forty. Her husband was an accountant and she had four children ranging in age from eighteen to eleven. She was admitted with a suspected cancer of the stomach which, it was believed, could be a secondary deposit from an earlier breast cancer for which she had had a mastectomy three years previously. When I interviewed her upon admission, Mrs Craig indicated that she herself suspected a connection between her past illness, which she knew to have been cancer, and her present condition.

> JM: What were you in for three years ago?
> Mrs C: What's the right word for the removal of my breast? Mastectomy I think they call it.
> JM: What was wrong with it?
> Mrs C: A puckering—not lumps or anything. It was cancer of course—the whole thing was removed.
> JM: Were you told it was cancer?
> Mrs C: Well they told me before the operation that if it was malignant they would have to remove the whole breast and when they did I knew that it was cancer. They wouldn't just hack it off for fun,

would they?

JM: Was the operation a success?

Mrs C: Well, yes, it has been a complete success—up to now, that is.

Later in the interview she revealed her suspicion that her present admission could be for treatment of 'a malignancy' and indicated clearly that, while she appreciated that the doctors could not give her a definitive answer at present, she wanted to know whether or not it was cancer when they had established the diagnosis.

JM: What are you in for now?

Mrs C: I can't tell you that nor can the doctors. I've got a tiny lump in my abdomen and it might be adhesions or fibroids but they're going to operate to find out. You see, once you've had cancer and go back to the doctor they're so careful. It might come back.

JM: Would you like to know what it is?

Mrs C: Oh yes. If it's cancer I want to know. There's no point in beating about the bush. People are frightened of the word 'cancer'—it's silly. They whisper it, 'she's had cancer.'

JM: How did you know anything was wrong?

Mrs C: What, this time or last?

JM: Well, both.

Mrs C: Well last time I read an article in a woman's magazine—it was about breast cancer—and it said that puckering was one of the signs so, as I had something that seemed to be similar, I thought I'd better go to the doctor. This time I just had a pain.

'Immediately' on feeling the pain she consulted her GP who told her that 'considering her case history' he would refer her to the consultant. He did not venture a diagnosis and she did not ask. When she saw the surgeon she was told that he could not, at that time, say what it was, it could be fibroids or 'adhesions', and that she would have to come into hospital for observation. Once in hospital, Mrs Craig was told that an operation was necessary in order to find out what her condition was and to help the doctors to decide what was to be done. At that point, and for the first time, she asked if she had cancer.

Mrs Craig: Is it a cancer, doctor?

Mr Donald: Well, I can't make statements like that at this stage. We'll have to do the operation to find out. But, if there's anything malignant about it, we might have to give you some additional treatment.

Investigations during the operation revealed that the growth was indeed malignant. When the doctors informed her of what they had done she repeated her question. This elicited a standard routine response which stopped short of the whole truth.

Mr Donald: Well Mrs Craig, there was a lump of fatty tissue on your stomach wall and inside it we found a swelling. When we removed the swelling and had a look at a bit of it under the microscope we found that it was active so we removed the lump and the surrounding area.

Mrs Craig: Is it cancer?

Mr Donald: Well, we don't actually call it a cancer but, if it had not been removed, it would almost certainly have turned into one. That's why we took it out—to save you having any more trouble with it.

This reply only partly satisfied her. She remained unclear as to what the distinction was between activity, potential cancer and actual malignancy. I asked her what the doctors had said.

Mrs C: Well, I've had a part of fatty tissue removed from my stomach wall. That's as far as I understand although they do their utmost to explain to you I've found. They had found a swelling inside this fatty part in my tummy. They removed the swelling and found it was active. Oh, and all the surrounding area has been removed too.

JM: Are you happy with your treatment?

Mrs C: Very. I came in for observation. I was prepared to be pronounced clear or otherwise. I know enough about cancer to know it could have been either way.

JM: Was it clear?

Mrs C: Well, they seemed happy with it and said it wasn't actually cancer.

JM: Are you satisfied with what you've been told. . . ?

Mrs C: Most happy. Any questions I've asked have been answered and, I think, truthfully.

JM: You wanted the truth?

Mrs C: Yes.

JM: Did you want to know everything?

Mrs C: I wanted to know everything, yes.

JM: Did you ask what it was?

Mrs C: Yes.

JM: What did he say?

Mrs C: He answered truthfully—that they found this swelling.

JM: Was it malignant?

Mrs C: He said it was 'active'. I said, 'Is that a cancer?' He said, 'We don't actually call it a cancer but it might turn into one.' I don't know what the difference is.

JM: The difference?

Mrs C: Between being a cancer or being active or turning into a cancer.

JM: But it isn't cancer?

Mrs C: Well I don't know exactly. They just said it was active and would have turned into a cancer. Mr Donald said that if it was malignant I might get additional treatment. I didn't, so that's a good sign.

JM: So, is that it all fixed now?

Mrs C: Oh, I don't know about that. I hope so. I'm not going to ask about that. They probably couldn't say anyway. I'm just hoping for the best.

JM: Are you worried about anything then?

Mrs C: Well, whether it's been a success. I just hope it has.

Mrs Craig wanted to know if she had cancer and sought to find out by asking. But, while she wanted to know the truth, she did not receive a completely truthful answer. Nevertheless, she remained sceptical of it and was not entirely convinced that she did not have the disease. The diagnosis remained equivocal for her. The information which she had received still retained an element of threat. She had not been told categorically that she did not have cancer and this may well have been the source of doubt in her mind. Her attitude towards her prognosis was a different matter. She did not appear to desire information relating to it and certainly did not seek it directly. The fact that she had received no additional treatment was interpreted by her as being a hopeful sign and, while far from certain that she was cured, she hoped that this was the case. Any attempt to establish the validity of that hope could have threatened its retention.

Mr Hamilton was a sixty-seven year old widower who lived with his daughter and son-in-law. His only previous admission to hospital had been with a heart attack. On this occasion he was admitted with a suspected epithelioma in his left cheek. The growth had been present for six months before he had consulted his GP. At first he thought that it might have been caused by his false teeth, to which he also attributed the fact that he was plagued by mouth ulcers. 'Well, I've always had ulcers since those plastic teeth. Then this lump started.'

By his own admission, he was reluctant to visit the doctor with it and only went along when his daughter 'told' him to make an appointment. ('She thought it might be cancer you see.') By the time he saw his GP his suspicions were already aroused.

To tell you the truth, I was beginning to think it was cancer. It could be a cancer. So I said to the doctor, I said, 'It's cancer.' He said, 'I suppose it might be but it's not a deadly one if it is. I'll have to get better advice and you'll have to go into hospital to get it seen to.'

Within a week he was seen by the consultant. 'He didn't say what it was. He just said that it would have to be dealt with and that they would either take it out or give me injections or needles to shrink it.' He did not ask for a diagnosis when he was seen as an outpatient but the fact that he had to come into hospital alarmed him greatly. He interpreted this as indicating that his condition must be relatively serious. 'I was terrified. I thought to myself, "cancer of the throat."'

A fortnight later he was admitted to the ward. I saw him on the afternoon of his admission.

JM: What's the trouble?
Mr H: Mouth ulcers and there's a lump in the side of my mouth. I don't know what you'd call it. They have a name for it but I can't remember. They're going to take a bit of it off and send it away for investigation.
JM: Did they say anything about the treatment you would get?
Mr H: What is it they do for cancer? Radio. . .what is it? *I* say cancer but I haven't been told that.
JM: Would you like to be told if it was?
Mr H: Yes. I've had a coronary and learned to live with that. I wouldn't like to be told in advance that I was going to have cancer though. I don't know if they'll tell me if it's malignant but I'd like to know.

So, upon admission, Mr Hamilton strongly suspected that he had cancer and said he wanted to know. A biopsy was planned and he was told that, depending upon the result of it, they 'might put some needles into the growth in order to shrink it.' The biopsy was duly performed but investigation of the sample took five days to complete. During that time, whether or not he was to get the 'needles' was a great source of worry for him. If this method of treatment was employed he would interpret it as an indication that the biopsy had shown that he had cancer.

> Mr H: They've taken a bit away to see if it was malignant. If it is then I'll get these needles. Mr Thomson (a fellow patient) says they're radium needles.
> JM: Have you asked if it's malignant?
> Mr H: Not yet. But, if I get the needles, I'll know it's cancer.

However, while he would take an implant as meaning that he had cancer, this was tempered, in some measure, by a conversation which he had with a district nurse relative of his. She had told him that if he was getting radium needles it meant that the growth was localised. 'That took a load off my mind', he said. So, while the implant would still be taken to mean that he had a malignancy, (this was implicit in what his relative had said), at least it would also indicate that it was localised. He was to cling to this for the rest of his eventful stay in the ward.

The day after his conversation with the district nurse, his daughter came to see him and, according to the resident, told him that his GP had told her that he had cancer. He, in turn, faced the resident with this news. I did not witness the encounter but the resident reported to me that Mr Hamilton had told him what his daughter had allegedly said and asked him if it was true. The resident reassured him that this was not necessarily the case and that, even if it was, the public's conception of cancer as being tantamount to a death sentence was misleading and at variance with the truth. He went on to explain that there were many different types of malignancy, with different degrees of virulence, some of which were eminently curable, and that the term 'cancer' was therefore a misleading one to apply. Mr Hamilton told me later that 'he (the doctor) sat for ages and explained that it wasn't cancer'. He could not recall the details of what he was told but he was certainly reassured.

Eventually the biopsy report arrived in the ward. It was negative. The resident informed him of the result. 'The results of the test on that were normal. There was no sign of any cancerous cells being present.'

Then an interesting thing happened. After displaying his relief at that news—'Oh, I'm glad to hear that', Mr Hamilton apologetically admitted that his GP had not said that he had cancer. 'I made a mistake earlier doctor. My doctor didn't say that I had cancer he just told my daughter that I had a growth and I read between the lines. A growth only meant one thing to me—a cancer.'

This raises an intriguing, but unfortunately unanswerable question. Had he said that he had been told that he had cancer as a tactic to get at the truth, or did he genuinely believe that the term 'growth' was synonymous with 'cancer'? However, that apart, Mr Hamilton was elated at having received such good news. 'I'm delighted. He told me it wasn't malignant.' Meanwhile, however, the doctors were having second thoughts and were not convinced of the accuracy of the biopsy report which appeared to conflict with the clinical evidence. They did not quite trust the report while the clinical signs were suggestive of malignancy. The matter was brought up at the ward conference where the surgeon in charge of the case expressed the opinion that, even if the results were negative at present, he believed that the growth was about to go malignant and that, consequently, it should be treated accordingly. It was decided that a second biopsy should be performed and that, irrespective of its result, they should probably proceed with the radium implant on the basis of the clinical evidence alone. Mr Hamilton was duly informed of this revision in policy.

> Now Mr Hamilton, the report we got back on that was negative but we won't take that on its own when the clinical signs were that something should be done. We could let you go home with it and you might be back in two months with it a lot worse. So we'll take another biopsy—you won't feel anything, you'll get a general anaesthetic this time—and then we'll have a chat about it to see what's to be done.

Mr Hamilton was clearly depressed at this news and as the consultant left his bedside the resident approached him and said reassuringly, 'It's nothing to worry about—it's just to make sure.' He replied, 'Oh, you're better to make sure.' We left him looking very depressed.

On the day he was to go to theatre he was again reassured, this time by the surgeon, that he did not think that he had 'anything to worry about' and that the investigation was being repeated purely as a safeguard. He inquired if the results would 'take five days like the last one' and was told that they would 'freeze it on the spot and get the result there and then.' The implant was carried out that afternoon although the biopsy report was again negative. I spoke to Mr Hamilton briefly on the following morning.

Well, they've given me the needles as you can see. But I haven't got the result of the test yet. I haven't asked them for it and I'm not goint to ask. I think it's best not to ask. I think they've got it local-ised though—at least, that's what I hope.

His remarks revealed the assumption that the result of the biopsy must have been positive and that he therefore had a malignancy. Other-wise, why would they have carried out the treatment? But, while he assumed that it was probably cancer, he indicated that he would rather retain the hope that the lesion was localised than ask questions relating to extent of involvement and the outlook for the condition. Later that morning he was informed that the biopsy had again been negative. 'The test we got yesterday was negative. It was just as dubious as the first one but we went ahead and did the operation just in case.'

Mr Hamilton was by now thoroughly confused. Apparently he did not have cancer but then, if he did not, why did they carry out the treat-ment. He now had two strong and conflicting pieces of information to contend with and somehow to reconcile. He voiced his puzzlement when I saw him together with his neighbour in the ward, Mr Wright.

Mr H: I can't understand it. They did one test and got clearance and did another and got clearance again but they did the operation all the same. I don't know if it's cancer or not. They said it wasn't but I don't know.

At this point Mr Wright interjected, 'They did it just to be on the safe side.'

Mr Hamilton was not convinced. The only way in which he could make sense of such apparently contradictory information was to inter-pret it as meaning that he was being experimented upon. For him this was the only plausible explanation for having received the treatment if he did not have cancer and he replied, 'Well, so they say. But I think they're experimenting with me. If the tests were negative, why else would they do the operation?'

Thereafter, there was no point in his asking if he had cancer as he had been virtually told that he did not. He did not enquire further. However, the fact that he had received the treatment aroused a suspicion which could not be completely dispelled. Nevertheless, his residual fear that he might have cancer was tempered by the hope that, at least, it was probably localised. Confusion over his diagnosis and why he had received the implant was still in evidence when I interviewed him on discharge. The belief that the treatment had been carried out as a safeguard, as he had been informed, and the idea that he was an unconscious party to an experiment, vied for superiority as acceptable explanations of the apparently contradictory nature of what had happened to him. This was never resolved.

> Mr H: I twice had a biopsy. The first came back negative then when
> I went to get the needles in they took another piece and put the
> needles in. It came back negative as well. It was heartening for
> me that they were making doubly sure by putting the needles in.
> (Pause.) But I couldn't get over them putting in these needles when
> the result was negative. Maybe they were experimenting on me.
> But I still don't understand why they gave me the needles know-
> ing it was negative.
> JM: Are you happy with your treatment then?
> Mr H: Oh yes. Very happy. Well, they leave nothing to chance.
> JM: Was the treatment what you had expected?
> Mr H: I didn't know what to expect. But I took it in my head that it
> must be cancer. I thought, 'Cancer of the throat'. I thought to
> myself, 'If they give me the needles, I'll know it was cancer'. But
> they gave me the needles and said it wasn't.
> JM: Did you want to know?
> Mr H: I wanted to know. Yes.
> JM: Are you satisfied with what you've been told.
> Mr H: Yes. I wanted to know and I think they told me.

Mr Hamilton had wanted to know the truth about his diagnosis and had, in fact, received it. While he was unable to completely resolve the apparent paradox of having received treatment while, at the same time, being informed that he did not have cancer, he was able to reconcile them in part by accepting the doctors' explanation that the treatment was a prophylactic measure and by, alternatively, explaining it in terms of experimentation. But, even then he was not entirely convinced that he did not have cancer and sought comfort in the qualifying belief that, even if he did, it was localised.

Patients who Suspected their Diagnosis and both wanted Confirmation of it and Information about their Prognosis

There were six patients in this group. They both desired, and sought to obtain, information on their diagnosis and prognosis. However, although

the following patients wanted some indication of the outlook for their
condition, they did not want to know whether or when they were likely
to die. Rather, what they required was some assessment of the extent of
involvement of the disease and a statement as to whether or not it had
been contained. Consequently, while these patients asked a number of
questions relating to the progress and possible course of their illness, no
patient asked if he was going to die.

Mrs Wilson was a forty-one year old mother of three whose husband
worked as a company representative. She was admitted with a suspected
carcinoma of the breast. She had consulted her GP shortly after detecting the lump because, as she said, 'I'm always pretty cautious about
things like that.' Her GP 'didn't say anything' and referred her to the
specialist 'to see what it is'. A week later she was seen by the consultant
surgeon and reported the following conversation with him: 'He said, "If
I told you there was nothing there I'd be telling you a lie because there
is a bit of thickening." Then I asked him if it was serious and he said
he couldn't tell me "till they did some tests."'
  A month elapsed between her outpatient appointment and her
admission to the ward and she confessed that her eventual admission
had come as a relief to her. 'I don't think I could have waited too long
or I would just have got more worried.'
  I interviewed her on the day following her arrival in the ward. She
was clearly aware that she could have cancer and stated that she wanted
to know. She indicated further that, if it transpired that she did have a
malignancy, her main concern would be to establish what the outlook
was.

JM: What's the trouble Mrs Wilson?
Mrs W: Something in my breast but I just don't know what it is. My
    sister had a breast lump. But I'm not necessarily worried that it's
    a lump like hers because it isn't that sort of lump. Mine is just a
    flat patch.
JM: Are you worried about it?
Mrs W: Well, the sooner they find out what it is the better it'll be. I
    want to know if it's what my sister had.
JM: What did she have?
Mrs W: She had her breast off. It was cancer. If I have cancer I'll want
    to know if I'm clear of it.
JM: Will you ask?
Mrs W: Yes I'll ask.

Mrs Wilson was to find herself involved in a lengthy campaign to ascertain the nature of her condition and its prognosis. At first she was informed that a number of investigations had to be conducted in order 'to find out what it is'. She was then subjected to a series of X-rays, mammograms and other tests. These proved inconclusive. She was informed that, while a firm diagnosis had not been reached, she would nevertheless require an operation.

> We've got the result of your X-rays but we'll still have to take more tests. To be quite honest, we just don't know what it is. But it will require an operation—there's no doubt about that. But we'll take more tests first because we like to know as much as possible before we operate.

Mrs Wilson felt that the difficulty in reaching a diagnosis could be a good sign. She sought confirmation of this on the following day.

> Dr Craib: We're still not sure about the results of your tests.
> Mrs Wilson: Does this mean there's nothing there then?
> Dr Craib: Oh no. There's something there all right but we don't know if it's *serious* or not. We'll have to take some more tests because the treatment you get will depend on them. There is some activity there though and you will need an operation. But it's a good sign from your point of view that we haven't been able to find anything definite yet because it means that it's small and early.

So Mrs Wilson did not receive the reassurance which she sought and hoped for: that delay in diagnosis meant that she might not have cancer. On the contrary, she had been informed that she definitely had something which had to be treated and despite the euphemistic mode in which this information was imparted to her she was not convinced that this something was not a malignancy. Indeed, when the doctors left her bedside, she turned to her neighbour and said, 'That's their story.' As I followed the doctors to the next patient I was unable to hear the rest of the conversation. But when I spoke with her later that morning the reason for her scepticism was clear. 'I think what they really mean is it's a small and early *cancer*.' But, although she wanted to know if she had cancer, at that stage, with the doctor 'confessing' that he did not know the diagnosis, there was no point in Mrs Wilson asking for it. She resolved to reserve that question for later. While she revealed that she was 'anxious' about her condition, she had taken some comfort from what the doctor had told her and had revised her original hypothesis that delay in reaching a diagnosis could mean that she did not have cancer to the hope that delay might mean 'that it's not too serious'. It was decided that her operation should take place on the following Wednesday afternoon and she was informed of this. The surgeon spoke with her on the morning of her operation.

> Mr Moorhead: Well Mrs Wilson, we'll see you this afternoon then.
> Mrs Wilson: The sooner the better.
> Mr Moorhead: You're not nervous are you?
> Mrs Wilson: Yes I'm nervous. I want to know what it is—that's what I'm nervous about.

The growth was malignant and her breast was removed. The following morning she asked what had been found.

> Mrs Wilson: What did you find?
> Dr Craib: Well, in the middle of that thing there were a few suspicious cells so we took it away just to be sure. But it was very small, very small. It'll give you no more bother. But it's a good job you saw about it when you did. It's just as well we didn't ask you to come back in three year's time.

Although this latest communication did not persuade Mrs Wilson that she did, or did not, have cancer, the fact that her breast had been removed tended to confirm her suspicion that the growth must have been malignant. Having reached that tentative conclusion, she was now concerned to assess how bad it was. She decided that the best way of realising her objective of gauging the extent of involvement of the disease, and hence the possible outlook, was by establishing whether or not her operation was to be supplemented by radiotherapy.

> JM: What did you have done in the operation?
> Mrs W: I had my breast off. They said it was suspicious cells and that it was better that they took it away. Dr Craib said it was just as well that they didn't ask me to come back in three years.
> JM: Were you anxious before your operation?
> Mrs W: Well I can't say because I didn't know what they were going to do. If I had known I would have wondered how far it had gone and how bad it was. But I got a surprise when I found out they'd taken my breast off. I hadn't realized it was that serious. I just

wonder now if I'll get radiotherapy like my sister did.

JM: Have you asked about that?

Mrs W: No. I haven't got round to asking that yet.

JM: What do you mean when you say you hadn't realized it was serious?

Mrs W: Well, it was probably malignant. That's why they operated presumably.

JM: Why are you concerned about whether you'll get radiotherapy?

Mrs W: Well then I'll know how bad it is and how far it's advanced.

On the Saturday morning Mrs Wilson initiated the following exchange:

Mrs Wilson: Will I need any X-ray treatment after this doctor?' The doctor hesitated and she went on, 'You said you found some suspicious cells but was it malignant?

Dr Ogston: Well certainly if you hadn't come in when you did and if we hadn't taken it out it would have become malignant. But whether you get radiotherapy or not does not depend on the severity of it. It depends on other things like your age, your general condition, how much muscle was left after the operation and several other things. If there had been nothing suspicious about the lump we wouldn't have given you radiotherapy but, if it is at all suspicious, we might, depending on these other things. But it's not because it was bad that we'll give you treatment. However, whether you get treatment or not is Dr Shoemark's decision.

Mrs Wilson had evidently been suspicious of the term 'suspicious cells' and had determined to find out if this was an euphemism for cancer. She found the doctor's reply unconvincing.

Well, I asked him if it was malignant and he said it would have become malignant. But I'm pretty sure it was cancer. He didn't say it wasn't. They probably just didn't want to tell me. But I still don't know if I'm going to get radiotherapy. I asked Dr Ogston and he said it didn't depend on how serious it was and that it depended on a lot of other things like how much muscle they had to cut, my age and my general condition.

Two days later Mrs Wilson was told that she would not be receiving radiotherapy. She was delighted at this news. 'I got some goods news this morning. I'm not getting radiotherapy after all. That really gave me a lift. It showed me that it isn't as serious as I thought.'

So, despite what the doctor had told her, she had still been equating the receipt of radiotherapy with severity. Anyway, she was now greatly heartened and believed the prognosis to be good. I interviewed her again before she went home.

JM: How are you feeling Mrs Wilson?

Mrs W: I'm feeling all right. I'm glad to be going home. When they said that I didn't have to have treatment that bucked me up a bit. It couldn't have been as bad as I thought.

JM: What did you have done?

Mrs W: I had my breast taken off—cancer of the breast.

JM: Were you told that's what it was?

Mrs W: No. But I think it'd been cancer right enough.

JM: Why's that?

Mrs W: Well, despite what they say, they wouldn't have taken my breast away if it wasn't would they? Anyway, I'm glad I didn't get radiotherapy. That probably means that they got it in time. At least, I hope they did.

JM: If you had got radiotherapy, what would you have done then?

Mrs W: I'd have asked them how bad it was and how far it had spread. I just would have had to know.

JM: Are you happy with your treatment then?

Mrs W: Yes, very happy, although I was surprised when they took my breast off.

JM: But you think it's been successful?

Mrs W: Oh yes.

JM: Do you have to come back for anything?

Mrs W: Well, I'll have to come back for check-ups. But I would like to come back just to make sure everything is all right.

JM: What about what you've been told about your treatment and condition. Are you satisfied with that?

Mrs W: Yes I think so. If you ask they'll tell you but if you just lie there they won't tell you. They tell you everything you want to know if you ask. Some people say they don't like to ask but I've always found them very co-operative. I asked after the operation what it was. I wanted to know what it was. Then when they said I didn't have to have treatment I felt it couldn't have been quite as bad as I'd imagined after the operation.

JM: Are you still worried about anything?

Mrs W: Not since I got the results back and I'm not getting radiotherapy.

Mrs Wilson had wanted to know if she had cancer and had also wanted an assessment of her prognosis. She had sought to obtain these by asking. The worst period for her had been that immediately following her operation when the removal of her breast had suggested that she had cancer and when she was still highly uncertain and anxious about the prognosis. The news that she was not to receive radiotherapy had injected a measure of certainty and optimism into her view of the outlook. Upon her discharge from the ward, despite the doctors' attempts to deflect her growing awareness, she was virtually certain that she had cancer. After all, as she said, she had not been explicitly told that she did not have the disease and, as far as she was concerned, all the other signs pointed to her having a malignancy. However, this knowledge did not weigh too heavily upon her as she had taken the absence of radiotherapy to indicate that, irrespective of the diagnosis, the probable outlook was good. Her optimism was probably justified.

Mrs Reid was a fifty-four year old married woman. She had no children and worked in a City supermarket. She was admitted to Ward 4C with a suspected carcinoma of her left breast. After detecting the lump in her breast, she had delayed for eight months before consulting her doctor. She said she had not considered it to be important. 'Well, I thought nothing of it. There was no pain. Then I thought, "It's not going, so I'd better go." I thought I'd done it decorating or something you see.' Her GP referred her to the specialist without venturing a diagnosis. She did not ask him what it might be. I was in attendance at her outpatient consultation where, after examining her, the surgeon said, 'Well Mrs Reid, there's a thickening there. I can't say what it is at the moment. You'll have to come into hospital so that we can find out what it is and decide upon what sort of treatment we'll give you. But it will almost certainly require an operation.' Mrs Reid did not comment. But when I saw her later in the ward, I asked what she had thought about what the consultant had told her in the clinic.

> I was up to ninety-nine. I thought it was just a cyst I had but when he told me he thought I would need an operation that made it worse. It was the thought of getting it off. And I wondered if it was just there or if it was farther on than they were saying.

A month passed before she was admitted. She would have preferred to have come in earlier. 'Well, I was very worried about it. I couldn't sleep.' When I saw her upon her arrival in the ward she was very anxious and certainly suspected cancer. One cue which she had seized upon was the fact that she was in Ward 4C having learned of its significance during the course of her mother's admission. She was also very conscious that the disease, if it was cancer, could have spread.

> Mrs R: I've a lump in my left breast. I don't know what it is. It might be cancer but I don't know.
> JM: Are you worried about it?
> Mrs R: Very. I'm worried about where else it might have gone to. My mother was in this ward ten years ago and it didn't do her much good. (Her mother had died of cancer.)

Her anxiety increased when it was confirmed that she would have to have an operation and when she was warned that her breast might have to be removed.

> Well Mrs Reid, we've decided to take you to theatre tomorrow morning. We'll take a bit of that thing out and have a look at it under the microscope and, depending upon what we find, we'll either take the lump out or remove the whole breast. It might be a cyst but if it looks at all suspicious we'll remove your breast, and perhaps the underlying muscle too, just to be sure.

I asked Mrs Reid what she felt about her impending operation.

> Mrs R: Well, I'm worried about it. I'm anxious all right with the news I got. The surgeon thinks it'll have to come off. He explained that they would do a biopsy during the operation and if it's posit-ive they'll take the breast away and maybe some of the muscle too. Whether it's cancer or not I don't know. They'll find out tomorrow. I'm just hoping it's OK.
> JM: Did he say it might be cancer?
> Mrs R: No, he didn't say.
> JM: Would you like to know?
> Mrs R: I'd like to know, yes. I will know. It depends what they do to me. If they take it off I'll know it was cancer.

The lump was malignant and her breast was amputated. The surgeon saw her on the following morning.

> Now Mrs Reid, when we had a look at that thing under the micro-

scope there were some nasty cells which would almost certainly have become dangerous if we had left it. So we took your breast away just to be safe. You should be all right now though. I wouldn't worry about it.

True to what she had said, Mrs Reid interpreted the removal of her breast as meaning that the lump must have been malignant. Her main concern now was to find out if it had spread.

Mrs R: Well it must have been cancer. They took my breast off. But I'm worried if it has spread or not. I just don't know if it has spread or if they've nipped it in the bud.
JM: Will you ask about that?
Mrs R: Oh, I'll ask all right.

She was then informed that she might have to undergo a course of radio-therapy.

Dr Barron: Now Mrs Reid you won't be getting home just yet. We might give you some radiotherapy as a safeguard so that, if there are still some suspicious cells lurking about, the radiation will get them. This doesn't mean that your condition is worse than we thought at first—we would just do it as a. . .
Mrs Reid: Safeguard.
Dr Barron: Yes. Just to make sure.

This did nothing for her confidence in the outlook and she expressed the view that, if she did get radiotherapy, she would take it to mean that the disease had not been eradicated and that it had spread. 'He said I might get radiotherapy. If I do I'll know they didn't get it all.' However, the radiotherapy was not necessary and she was informed of this. 'Your tests were clear so we've decided not to give you radiotherapy.'
Mrs Reid was greatly heartened by this and interpreted it as being a good sign.

Mrs R: Well, Dr Chisholm told me the laboratory tests were all clear and I wouldn't need any radium treatment. That was a relief.
JM: Why was it a relief?
Mrs R: Well, I thought it had spread. I thought it was further on because it was eight months till I went to the doctor. I told you before that my mother was in here ten years ago for cancer, and

that's what worried me.

There then occurred an incident which demonstrated that, although greatly relieved by the news that she was not to receive radiotherapy and despite being told the tests were negative, she was not entirely convinced that she was clear of the disease. I was not present at the encounter but Mrs Reid reported that it went like this: 'I saw Dr Barron and I said to him, "Are you sure it's nowhere else?" He said, "Yes." Then I said, "You're just saying that", and he said, "Look", and he showed me a letter on the tests and it said "negative, negative, negative."'

By calling his honesty into question, Mrs Reid had apparently induced the consultant to show her the report on the investigations. She was now satisfied that the outlook was probably good and was much more relaxed when I interviewed her finally just before she went home.

JM: How are you feeling now Mrs Reid?

Mrs R: I'm feeling fine.

JM: What have you had done?

Mrs R: I had my breast removed. I thought it was a cyst but it couldn't have been. I got a fright when I heard that it was cancer.

JM: Did somebody tell you?

Mrs R: No, they never said. I just guessed.

JM: Did you expect the operation?

Mrs R: Well, they warned me but I wasn't expecting the operation I got, if you know what I mean. I thought it was a cyst. But I knew what to expect because a girl in the shop had a breast off and she told me about it.

JM: So you had known what to expect?

Mrs R: Well no, because I didn't think I'd the same. I thought I'd just a cyst.

JM: Are you satisfied with what you've been told?

Mrs R: Yes. I wanted to know if it was any farther and they told me it wasn't.

JM: Were you able to find out everything you wanted to know then?

Mrs R: Yes. They've really told me all that they could tell me.

JM: Are you at all worried about it now?

Mrs R: Well, not as worried as I was. I was worried if it had spread but I'm fine now that the tests were clear. You never know how far this has spread throughout your body and it was a relief after the operation that there were no more consequences to it.

JM: So you think you'll be OK now?

> Mrs R: I sincerely hope so. What more can I do but hope for the best?

On admission, Mrs Reid had suspected that she had cancer and had wanted to know if her suspicion was correct. Her arrival in Ward 4C had reinforced her fears. She took the removal of her breast as confirmation that she had cancer and thereafter sought to establish whether the disease had spread and thus to acquire some indication of the prognosis. This she did by asking and upon being assured that there was no other evidence of the disease she became reasonably, although not wholly, confident that she was clear.

Miss Edwards was a fifty year old secretary. She was admitted to Ward 4C with a lump in her right breast and another in her right armpit. She was highly aware that she could have cancer and it was this fear which had prompted her to consult her GP. She had, however, delayed for four months before doing so.

> Miss E: First I saw the lump under my arm and then I saw the one in my breast. But I thought nothing about it because I'd had it before and it went away.
>
> JM: How long had you had the lumps?
>
> Miss E: Oh, four months.
>
> JM: What finally persuaded you to see the doctor?
>
> Miss E: Well, it didn't go away and I've heard that it's dangerous and that it could be cancer and the sooner you go the better.

Her GP told her, 'We shouldn't take any chances with this. I think you should see the specialist.' She did not enquire of him what the diagnosis might be but when she saw the consultant she made a determined effort to find out if he thought it was cancer.

> When I saw Mr Moorhead he said there was something to come out. Then I put it to him, 'Have I cancer?' He said, 'You're putting me on the spot.' I said, 'Maybe, but it's your job. What do you think?' I said I didn't want any fairy stories. He said, 'I think so.' But, if I hadn't asked, he wouldn't have said. He said, 'I see you like to know things.' I said, 'It's best to know the truth.' So the shock's past for me. When they find it's bad, it won't be such a shock for me. And, of course, it's always at the back of my mind that it might not be. But I want to know. My brother died of cancer and everybody pretended that he didn't have it and that he was getting better.

I didn't like that. I think it's best to accept these things.

Two weeks later she was informed by telephone that arrangements had been made for her admission to the ward. The fact that she had been telephoned caused her some alarm. 'I thought, "Telephone. They're getting me in quick. It must be cancer."' Nevertheless, she was glad that she had been admitted so swiftly. 'The sooner it's over the better. There's less time to think about it.'

I interviewed her on the day after her admission.

Miss E: There's a lump in my breast and one under my arm. I'm not supposed to know what kind of lump it is. It could be bad and it might not be. But I think Mr Moorhead thinks it's bad. I just asked him point blank. And if you've got cancer they can't cure it can they? They can only keep you going for a while. But they'll probably have to do tests before they know for sure.

JM: What made you think it might be cancer?

Miss E: Because so many of these breast conditions are.

JM: Is it worrying you?

Miss E: Oh yes, I'm worried. Sometimes you forget and I'm all right. Next time I'm down.

Miss Edwards very decidedly wanted to know if she had cancer. She had asked and had been told that this was likely. But although she believed that this was probably the case, she still, at this stage, retained some hope that it might not be. However, if it were confirmed that she did have the disease, her conception of the prognosis for cancer appeared to be such as to afford her little hope for the outlook.

During her first few days in the ward, Miss Edwards underwent a series of investigations and on the fifth day she asked Dr Craib if it was cancer. He replied, 'Well we can't say yet but, if it is, it's slow growing. But we'll know about it after your operation on Tuesday.'

On the following day she was informed that her breast would have to be removed—'We've decided to take the whole breast away Miss Edwards, and some of the underlying muscle as well. That thing in your breast is certainly active and would be dangerous if it was left.'

She received a radical masectomy. There was no evidence of presence of the disease other than in her breast and axilla. After her operation she sought to establish, by asking, whether the growth had been malignant and if it was likely to recur.

> Mr Moorhead: Your operation went well yesterday. But in that lump
>   there were some nasty cells so we removed your breast and the
>   muscle underneath it as well otherwise there's no doubt it would
>   have given you trouble in the future.
> Miss Edwards: Was it cancer then?
> Mr Moorhead: Well yes, you could call it a cancer. But we got it all.
>   That's why we took away the glands and muscles as well.
> Miss Edwards: But it'll just come back somewhere else won't it?
> Mr Moorhead: Not necessarily. We certainly don't expect it to. You
>   see with the breast we can remove the whole thing. This isn't so
>   easy with somewhere like the stomach. But we expect you to be
>   all right now. So I wouldn't worry about it.

When I spoke to her on the same afternoon she was clearly reassured
by what she had been told.

> But the best was what he told me afterwards. I asked if it would
> come back somewhere else and he said, 'Not necessarily.' Wasn't
> that good news now. It has really taken a load off my mind. I would
> rather know the truth. If you think they're withholding information
> you might fear the worst and think they're not telling you because
> it's serious.

She asked no further questions during the remainder of her stay in
the ward. Through her persistence and her demand for the truth ('no
fairy stories'), Miss Edwards had obtained confirmation that she had
cancer from the consultant himself. He had also given her a truthful
answer to her questions about the possible prognosis. But when I interviewed her on the day before her discharge, while she still took comfort
from the reassurances which she had received after her operation, she was
not absolutely convinced that she was completely cured. She did not
entirely trust the doctor's assurances believing that he might simply
have been trying to spare her anxiety. In addition, even if he had been
telling her the truth as he saw it, she was not convinced that even *he*
could be certain that the disease would not recur. But while she went
home believing that there was a large question mark against her future,
above all, she did still *hope* that the disease would not reappear and
that she might be cured. Whereas initially she had believed the prognosis for cancer to be hopeless, she now had hope.

> JM: What sort of operation did you get?

Miss E: I had a mastectomy for cancer in my breast, a radical I think they call it, and a lump removed from under my arm. I think radical refers to roots. They didn't say it was cancer. It was me who mentioned cancer.

JM: What did they tell you about it?

Miss E: They told me everything's removed but whether that's the truth I don't know. They may be saying that to put my mind at ease. You see I thought when you had cancer it came back but they didn't see any reason that it should. They said that in the breast they can remove the whole thing but not in the stomach.

JM: Are you satisfied with what you've been told?

Miss E: Well yes, I kept asking. I don't suppose they would have told you if you didn't ask. But there again, maybe a lot of patients don't want to know so they have to treat them half and half so as not to scare them. All I wanted to know was if I was perfectly clear and apparently I am. I've been told that. And it won't come back anywhere else. I've been assured of that. I said to Mr Moorhead 'You're better to know.' I'd be more worried if I didn't know.

JM: Were you able to find out all you wanted to know by asking?

Miss E: I could have read between the lines but I wanted to make sure.

JM: Would you have reached the same conclusions by yourself?

Miss E: Yes, except for the final one. Will it come again? Which I suppose I can't expect anyone to answer one hundred per cent. But I expect they'll keep a hold of me for a few years for checkups. I'd rather they did that so they can catch it quickly if it does come back.

JM: Are you worried about anything now?

Miss E: The outcome. But my mind's at ease now. I think I can believe them.

JM: So you think you'll be OK?

Miss E: The only thing that I'm not sure if I can believe is if it won't break out again. But maybe they can't tell. Maybe no doctor could.

Mr Harvey, a thirty-nine year old labourer, was admitted with a suspected melanoma on his shin. He was single and lived in lodgings. He was definitely aware of the possibility that he could have cancer and wanted to find out. His GP had confirmed that his suspicion could be well founded. He was also very worried that he might lose his leg.

Mr H: I've got a mole thing on my leg. I just hope they don't take my leg off. If it's anything serious, cancer like, they might have to take my leg off. But they don't know what it is yet—not till they take it out and test it. But I've heard of people having cancer in their leg and having it taken off.

JM: How did you discover it?

Mr H: I just said to the doctor, 'I've got a funny thing on my leg.' I thought nothing of it.

JM: Why did you go to him with it?

Mr H: Well, you worry about things that grow and I showed some of my mates and they said they'd heard of moles turning into cancer. I'd heard about it myself.

JM: What did he say about it?

Mr H: Well, I said, 'What is it?' He said he didn't know. Then I said, 'Is it gangrene?' He said, 'No', so I said, 'Come clean, is it cancer?' He said he thought it might be. I got a shock then but I'm all right now.

JM: Did you ask the consultant what it was when you saw him?

Mr H: No. He said I would have to come in for tests and that they would remove it but he couldn't say what it was till they did tests on it.

JM: Do you want to know if it is cancer?

Mr H: Yes, I want to know. And I want to know if it's spread.

He was prepared for his operation in the following way: 'We're going to take this off. It will depend on the report we get on it whether we'll do anything else but if it's active we might take a bit away from around here too and give you a skin graft. But we're uncertain as to its real nature so we'll have a look at it under a microscope first.'

I talked to Mr Harvey just before his operation and he indicated that the type of operation which he received would inform him of the diagnosis.

JM: How do you feel about your operation today?

Mr H: Well, I've had operations before and they've never bothered me but I've been more worried about this one than any of them.

JM: Why?

Mr H: Well, with my own doctor thinking it might be cancer. If it has spread. . .well I don't know.

JM: Is it that it might have spread that worries you most?

Mr H: Yes. If they do the big operation, I'll know it's cancer and that it might have spread.

The biopsy report, received while he was in theatre, was equivocal and full confirmation, by means of a different test, could not be obtained for several days. But the clinical evidence suggested a strong possibility of malignancy so the mole was removed together with a sizeable area surrounding it. He also received the skin graft. He was told,

Well, Mr Harvey, we had a look at that thing under the microscope and it was certainly active so we took it away or it might have caused you bother in the future. We also took a fair bit from around it just to be on the safe side. But we've still to wait for the results of other tests until we know exactly what it was. We'll get them in a few days.

After the operation Mr Harvey had two main concerns: to establish with certainty whether he had cancer and, if so, to find out if it had spread. He made a determined effort to acquire answers to these questions. This was not easy. The fact that he was regarded by the medical staff as being 'agitated' and 'demanding', and might therefore react badly to being told explicitly that he had cancer, did not help his cause. On the second day after his operation he asked if the results of the tests had arrived and was told that they had not. He repeated his request on the following morning somewhat to the doctor's annoyance.

Mr Harvey: Are the results of the tests back yet?
Dr Ogston: No. You'll just have to be patient. I told you yesterday that there are a lot of them to do and we have to wait our turn.

Three days later he again asked about the tests. But the results had still not come through and he was told so. On the following morning the report on the biopsy arrived. Mr Harvey asked his usual question.

Mr Harvey: Have you got the report back yet doctor?
Mr Donald: Well yes, that was certainly active and would have been dangerous if we had left it there. There's none of it left though. That's why we did such a wide excision.

This did not satisfy him and he probed further.

Mr Harvey: But was it cancer?
Mr Donald: Well, if it hadn't been removed, it would certainly have become malignant. But we've got it all away.

Mr Harvey was still not satisfied. Next morning he again collared the surgeon and again he received an equivocal reply although this time it was conceded that he had 'a kind of cancer'.

Mr Harvey: You say it would have become malignant but is it cancer now? I want to know.

Mr Donald: Well, there was some activity there but I can't really put a name to it. I suppose you could call it a kind of cancer but there are lots of different sorts: some need further treatment and some don't. But you won't need any more treatment and there are no further deposits.

Mr Harvey: So, did you get it all?

Mr Donald: Oh yes. That's why we did such a wide excision—to make sure we got it all.

Mr Harvey: So there's none of it left is there?

Mr Donald: No. The tests which we did were all clear.

A little later, just for good measure, Mr Harvey asked the resident if it had been cancer and was told, 'I suppose you could call it a low-grade cancer. But we got it all. You've nothing to worry about.'

Persistence and a manifest determination to obtain the truth had won the day. While he was now resigned to the fact that he had obtained as much information as he was going to get, he now knew that he had had a cancer. Mr Harvey was satisfied. He had found out what he had wanted to know: he had had cancer but he believed that it had all been removed and that the prognosis was good.

Mr H: Well, I had a cancer in my leg but they got it all and I've no worries now.

JM: You're sure it was cancer?

Mr H: Positive. They said so. But not without a lot of pestering mind.

JM: And you've no worries now?

Mr H: None at all.

Nine months later he was admitted with secondaries.

Patients who knew that they had Cancer and wanted Information on their Prognosis

Each of the three patients in this group knew that they had a malignancy on admission to the ward. They sought to obtain information about the outlook for their condition. Like their predecessors, none of these patients wanted to be told explicitly that they were going to die.

Mrs Green was fifty-three, married to a tax inspector, had no children and was a diabetic. She was admitted with a sizeable lump in her left breast. She had been aware of its presence 'for a good few years' and had apparently not considered consulting her doctor with it because 'it never bothered me'. Her eventual consultation was precipitated by her reading an article on breast cancer in a woman's magazine when, she said, 'I got scared'. On her own admission, however, she had suspected cancer for a long time and suggested that this was the reason for her not going to her doctor sooner. 'Well, deep down I knew. Maybe that's how I kept putting it off. It was just really fear that kept me away before.'

She was also aware that cancer carried the risk of spread and this possibility was to become her main preoccupation during the course of her hospitalization. When she saw her GP he gave no opinion on the possible diagnosis and promptly referred her to the specialist because, he said, 'it has to be seen to'. The consultant was no more revealing in what he told her. 'He just said, "We'd better have you in and have the different tests carried out."'

However, her knowledge of his specialization in malignant diseases suggested to her that she had cancer. 'I knew when I saw Mr Donald that it must be cancer. You see, I know he's a cancer specialist.'

In a matter of days she was admitted to the ward. The consultant had contrived to neutralise any potential threat inherent in the speed of her admission. 'He said that there was a cancellation and that there was room for me.'

But, her admission to Ward 4C, with her attendant awareness of its primary function, confirmed the process of realization and reinforced her conviction that she must have cancer. 'Well, I know it's cancer. That's why I'm in here. This is the cancer ward.'

Having settled in her own mind that she had cancer, her main concern was to ascertain whether the disease had spread and whether the chances of success in the treatment of her condition were good.

Mrs G: All I'm worried about now, and all I want to know, is if it's spread and if they can cure me. But I have every confidence that they can do something for me.
JM: Would you like to know about these things?
Mrs G: Yes, I would like to know what's going to happen and to be told the truth. I don't like people beating about the bush.

In this context, she expressed a preference for having her whole breast removed rather than just having the lump taken out. That, she felt, would give her a greater measure of insurance against a recurrence. I'd rather they took the whole thing off than just take out the lump. If they take it off, I'll know it's all away but, if they just take out the lump, I'd worry in case it started up again.'

Her wish, if it can be called such, was granted. Having been prepared for the possibility in the usual way, she underwent a radical mastectomy. On the following day, the surgeon explained what he had done. Mrs Green made a determined effort to find out if she was 'clear'.

Mr Donald: Now Mrs Green, there were some suspicious cells in that lump so we took the whole breast off and cut away some of the underlying muscle.

Mrs Green: You got it all then?

Mr Donald: Yes.

Mrs Green: Are you sure it's all clear now?

Mr Donald: Oh yes. That's why we took the whole breast off and took the muscle away too—to make sure we got it all.

She derived great comfort from this encounter.

JM: What did the doctors say to you this morning?

Mrs G: I had my left breast removed complete. You call it a radical operation.

JM: What was it?

Mrs G: It'd been cancer.

JM: Did you ask that?

Mrs G: I didn't need to. I knew. But I asked if I was clear and he said I was. I'm very glad I asked. I don't care how long I've to stay in now as long as I'm clear. The scan worried me a lot. I was up to ninety in case they found anything else. But they say they haven't, so that's good.

However, later that same day, the skeletal survey, which had been carried out prior to her operation, revealed that she had multiple bone metastases. The scan had, as she said, alarmed her at the time and, indeed, before her operation she had expressed concern that her bones might be involved. At that stage there had been no reason to believe that this was so and when she had said, 'I hope there's nothing wrong with my bones', she had been told, 'Oh no. It's just a routine thing.' Now they certainly were involved and it was decided to treat her with drugs. This additional treatment was 'sold' to her in terms of 'making sure'. But, given that she feared spread of the disease and believed that *this* could be the reason for the additional treatment, this explanation did not satisfy her. In terms of her hope for the outlook, she was back at square one. 'They say I'm all clear then they give me more treatment. I just don't understand it. Maybe I'm not clear after all. . .I'm worried sick about it.'

It was not until she had been receiving injections for several days that she made her move. She refused an injection. She had been told that she would receive five injections and, having had them, she now wondered why the treatment was being extended. The Senior House Officer went to see her and walked into the following question.

> Mrs Green: I've been asking about the injections. I thought that when I'd had five I was finished. Does this mean that I'm not all clear?
> Dr Craib: No, not at all.
> Mrs Green: But I thought that when this was removed I'd be clear. Does this mean it's not all clear?
> Dr Craib: Oh no, it's just a precaution. We're just doing it as a safeguard. You'll agree that the more safeguards we can build into a system the better. We can use a combination of an operation, injections and radiation.
> Mrs Green: Oh well. I hope you don't think I'm being awkward. I just thought I'd ask before I took the injection but it's been explained to me now.

She appeared to accept this, although with reservations. 'Well, they still say I'm clear and that I'm just getting the injections as a precaution. I just hope that's the truth.'

In fact it was not the truth but Mrs Green was never to discover this while she was in hospital. The final incident occurred during the following week when it was decided to stop the injections for a while until her blood recovered from one of their side effects. The explanation for temporary cessation of the treatment provoked in Mrs Green a fear that she might have leukaemia.

> Dr Shoemark: We've decided to stop your injections for a bit Mrs Green because they're making your blood a bit thin. But we'll start them again when it recovers.

Mrs Green: Does this mean there's something wrong with my blood?
Dr Shoemark: Oh no. It's just the effect of the drug.
Mrs Green: It doesn't mean I've got anything like leukaemia does it?
Dr Shoemark: No, no. You've got nothing like leukaemia. As I say, it's just the effect of the drug.

Three weeks later Mrs Green completed her course of treatment and I saw her as she was preparing to go home. Having persistently sought to find out about the prognosis, and having received optimistic responses to her enquiries, Mrs Green was now relatively hopeful about the outlook. However, an element of doubt did still remain. The most encouraging sign for her had been when her husband had been given the same optimistic assessment as herself. This had served to reduce her reservations on the verity of what the doctors had told her although it did not eliminate them entirely. I asked if she considered that her treatment had been successful.

Mrs G: Well, they say it has been a success and I just hope so. My husband asked and he came and told me what they had told him and it was word for word what they had told me. I was really pleased with that.
JM: What did they tell him?
Mrs G: That I was clear. I thought they might tell him a different story. I thought they might tell him *the truth* but not me. So I'm keeping my fingers crossed that everything's really OK.[1]
JM: Were you able to find out all you wanted to know?
Mrs G: Yes. I wanted to know everything and I asked. Mind you, sometimes it wasn't too easy to find out. But I found them very willing to answer questions.
JM: Are you worried about the lump now?
Mrs G: Well it's away now. They said they got the whole lot out but here's hoping they did. I have to attend a clinic for a period. They like to keep a check on patients who've had cancer.
JM: Are you not sure that you'll be all right?
Mrs G: Well, I can't be altogether sure. You see, I'm not sure they told me all they could tell me. But they say I'll be all right and I just hope they're right. It might still kill me. (laughs)
JM: Would you like to know if it was going to? (lightheartedly)
Mrs G: No, not really. I don't think I'd like to go that far. I

don't think many people would like to be told they were going to die.

Note

1. Her husband had enquired about the position immediately following her operation and before it was known that she had metastases.

10 THE INFORMAL NETWORK

One potentially important source of information for patients remains to be discussed: the informal network. It was possible that patients could have obtained information from this quarter whether they wanted to know or not. The informal network consisted of relatives, fellow patients and a number of other people, excluding the medical and nursing staff, with whom the patients were in contact while in hospital.

Relatives and other hospital workers did not appear to play a significant part in supplying patients with information about their illness. Their relatives told them very little, if anything, that was unfavourable and certainly did not communicate their diagnosis to them.[1] On the other hand, they very swiftly conveyed any hopeful information which they had received to the patients. But this was usually no more than the patient himself had been told or had been able to find out. Nevertheless, the fact that somebody else had been told the same thing did serve to reinforce their faith in the optimistic reassurances which they themselves had received. What relatives might have transmitted to patients through their general demeanour and behaviour in their presence I cannot say.

Ancillary hospital workers, such as cleaners and porters, did not furnish the patients with significant information either. They were not asked for any and did not volunteer it. Patients did ask them about more mundane matters but perhaps their illness was thought to be too serious a question to discuss with them. The patients also believed that those workers could not possibly be in possession of what they wanted to know about their condition. Nor did the clergy, physiotherapists, radiographers or social workers appear to provide patients with information on the nature of their condition. Certainly no patient confessed to having received, or sought, information about their condition from any of them. Fellow patients were a different matter.

On both the male and female wards two distinct groups were perceived by the cancer patients. In the women's ward they saw a clear division between themselves and the gynaecology patients while on the male ward the dental patients were regarded as separate.

Well, there are two groups in the ward really. There's us, and we've all got the same sort of trouble. Then there's another group who are part of the ward yet not part of the ward; the gynaecology group. They're in for a different sort of thing.

This distinction was made whether the patients perceived their own part of the ward as comprising cancer patients or not. Apart from the fact that they had different types of condition from the other groups, their separateness was emphasized by their occupation of different parts of the ward and their treatment by different sets of doctors. Most cancer patients, however, did also see their own group as being composed of patients who had, at least, a suspected malignancy. 'There are the gynae patients at the other end and us at this end. It's a happy group at this end. We've something in common—our illness. We're all cancer patients up this end.'

Conversely, the other groups on the wards knew that they were sharing them with cancer patients—'They're all cancer patients up that end.' —and also regarded their own groups as being separate from them. This sense of separateness which was experienced by both groups, resulted in interaction between the cancer patients and the other groups on the wards being very limited. Although they did interact, the dominant pattern was for the two groups to keep themselves to themselves.

Among the cancer patients, in the context of their shared identity, there were no barriers to interaction; they all mixed freely. Thus, while they interacted only to a limited extent with the other groups on their wards, there was constant interaction among the cancer patients themselves and, insofar as this was the case, they saw their part of the ward as comprising one large group. 'We were just one big group. You wouldn't stay in one group all the time. Everybody made friends with everybody else. We all just go round speaking to one another. Nobody's left out.'

However, while it is true that the cancer patients constituted one group insofar as they interacted freely with one another and either perceived themselves as sharing a common identity as cancer sufferers or regarded themselves as being in some other sense separate from the others with whom they shared the ward, within this larger group certain subdivisions were apparent. Particular friendships and close associations were formed. There were two types of sub-group: friendship groups, and groups which were formed by patients for the specific purpose of discussing their illness. Thus, while each cancer patient would interact with every other in the context of the total ward group, each patient was also a member of particular friendship or discussion groups. A number of factors were involved in determining which patients grouped together. These varied greatly in their significance. In the friendship

groups, apart from a tendency for patients who were admitted to the
ward around the same time to group together: 'It's more easy to make
friends that way; coming in with people. We're all strangers together,'
there were no other consistent binding factors. Certainly, factors such
as age, common interests and whether patients came from the same
town or area played a part in the formation of friendships, but the
closest and most permanent associations on the ward emerged in response
to the sort of affinity which leads to the formation of any friendship. 'It's
just a matter of who's your cup of tea.' There was no evidence that having a similar condition led to the forging of special friendship bonds any
more than did other factors. On the other hand, similarity of condition
or treatment, and a willingness to discuss them, were central to the formation and composition of the groups in which the patients' conditions
were the topic of discussion.

These sub-divisions, or patient groupings, were fluid and overlapping.
The composition of the groups was constantly changing; members
would be discharged or would change groups and new patients would
join. Patients could also belong to more than one friendship group and
could move freely between them. Similarly, patients would discuss different aspects of their condition with different people. They might also
discuss their condition with different groups at different times according
to the contribution which they felt they could make to their understanding of what was happening at a particular stage of their treatment. Thus,
a patient who had to undergo a course of radiotherapy following a mastectomy might forsake fellow mastectomy patients as her prime discussion group in preference to others who were in receipt of the same treatment. Finally, patients would be members of friendship and discussion
groups simultaneously which meant that the membership of the two
types of group usually overlapped. However, many patients were not
members of discussion groups and it is the distinction between them
and those who were that I now wish to consider.

Those patients who did not take part in groups which discussed their
illness were generally those who did not want to have their diagnosis
confirmed and/or to find out about their prognosis. They did not participate in those groups for the same reasons that they did not question
the ward staff or seek to find out about their condition in other ways.
They did not want to know. Those patients who did not want to discuss
their illness made their feelings quite clear when I talked to them—'I
never discussed my condition although there's some patients who talk
about it all the time. I don't want to talk about it, and I don't. It's my
private concern and I'm not nosy about their troubles either.'

Thus, the discussion groups were made up entirely of patients who wanted to find out about their condition. For them, their fellow patients were simply another potential source of information. Of course, all patients, irrespective of whether or not they wanted to find out about their condition, discussed illness in terms of how they felt, what treatment they were going to get and, at a superficial level, what was wrong. The difference lay in the depth of discussion. The more general ones amounted to little more than asking and responding to, 'How are you?' and 'What are you having done?' The others were much more concerned with more detailed questions and the interpretation of events: was it malignant?; did the tests mean that it had spread?; would it come back? and so on. These were the sorts of discussions that some patients preferred to avoid because participation in them would have carried the risk of learning something that they would rather not know. In addition, talk about illness could be depressing. To have the disease, or to suspect that one had it, was bad enough but to be constantly talking about it would have been more than some patients could stand. 'With what I've got, if everybody's talking about their illness, I find it depressing. I couldn't tolerate it. I don't want to hear them talking about it spreading or coming back.'

Fortunately, those patients who wished to discuss their illness were not insensitive to the wishes of those who did not. They accordingly tended to confine such discussions to the company of a few like-minded patients. This usually succeeded in avoiding the situation where a patient found himself caught up in a discussion in which he had no desire to participate. However, patients were not always so tactful and, while discussion of illness was usually reserved for the appropriate settings, the overlapping nature of the ward groupings meant that the topic could occasionally be raised in inappropriate contexts. This could cause considerable consternation among patients who wished to avoid the subject and could even arouse outright hostility. There were a number of ways in which they attempted to handle the unwelcome raising of the topic of illness. Of course, if they found themselves in a group which was clearly intent upon discussing the matter, they could simply leave it. Approaches made to them individually could be more difficult to handle. Most patients would have the subject broached with them at some time. Apart from anything else, it was the only way in which others could ascertain whether or not they wished to discuss it. When this happened, they would gently let the other party know that they had no desire to talk about it. This might entail giving a limited reply to a question or not answering it at all.

> I never discuss it with anybody. They ask me what was the matter
> and I say, 'I had an operation and that's all I can tell you.' I don't
> encourage them. I let them know I don't want to talk about it.

> If they ask what I'm in for, I pretend I can't quite hear or smile
> broadly and ask how they're keeping.

Other patients usually got the message. But, even when a patient had
indicated that he did not want to talk about it, some patients might persist in trying to involve them in such discussions. This obliged patients
who were put upon in this way to adopt stronger measures in order to
discourage the persistent offender. They might change the subject
abruptly and in such a way as to indicate, in no uncertain terms, that
they did not wish to pursue the topic. They might stubbornly refuse to
answer questions or to comment upon the other patient's remarks about
his own condition. Or, they might just ignore him or even, as a last
resort, walk away.

> Mr Black keeps talking about how he's worried in case they find
> anything else. He mentions that about four times a day. I'm really
> fed up with it. I don't want to talk about it. I just try to ignore him
> and that seems to work. But I don't like doing it because it's rude to
> ignore people.

> She would keep on talking about her illness and it got up my back.
> So I just ignore her now when she talks about it. She usually stops
> then. But some of the others are as bad and I don't like discussing ill-
> ness. I try to avoid it. You can just go away if you can walk.

In conjunction with these deterrent measures, patients might also
attempt to minimise the damage which such loquacious individuals
could do to them. Quite simply, from the point of view of the patient
who did not want to find out about his illness, the less those patients
who persisted in talking about it knew the better, especially if they
were going to report everything they found out to them. Much unwanted
information could be received in this way. They would, therefore, occasionally attempt to dissuade the persistent patient from finding out
more about his own condition, or about the disease in general, by trying
to discourage him from questioning the staff or seeking information in
other ways, (as far as I could establish, this met with little success:)
'You'll only worry yourself if you keep trying to find out things.' 'Don't

go bothering the doctors by asking questions all the time.' 'Don't be so nosy.'

But not even all patients who sought to find out about their condition participated in discussions about illness. Some of them did not regard their fellow patients as being appropriate sources of information believing that their knowledge was likely to be inaccurate,—'I didn't discuss it with them because they didn't know. They were only guessing.' They therefore tended to avoid discussion of the topic. Still others, while not wishing to talk about their own condition for the same reason, were, however, prepared to listen to others and to comment upon what they had to say.

> Well, I didn't see any point in discussing my condition with them. They don't know anything about it. I'd rather just ask the doctors who do know. That way I can be sure of getting accurate information. But, if they want to talk about their troubles, you listen and tell them what you think. You try to reassure them.

While a large number of patients avoided discussions about illness, this did not mean that they remained ignorant of what was wrong with other patients in the ward. On the contrary, most patients were well aware that the others had a malignancy.[2]

> Well, it filters through to you what they've got. You get to know what everybody has, whether it's major or minor. I can tell you what's wrong with every patient in the ward. Murray has a cancer in his mouth, Mr Rees has one in his stomach, Ben Knight has a cancer in his jaw. . .

This was especially so with those who wanted to find out about their condition, but even those patients who wished to deny that they themselves had cancer were usually aware that this is what the other patients had. Of course, part of the reason they did not want to take part in the discussions was that they knew that their fellow patients had cancer and would be discussing the disease. The existence of this knowledge about other patients' conditions might appear to be incompatible with the hope that one did not have the disease oneself. However, it was one thing to reach that conclusion about others and quite another to confirm it for oneself. The deduction that one had the disease oneself did not follow inevitably from the conclusion that this is what the others had. It was always possible for a patient to maintain the belief that he might not have cancer even if most of the others on the ward did: 'Most of the others have cancer you know. I just hope I don't have it too.' His case might be an exception.[3] Patients who did not want to have their diagnosis confirmed were at pains to establish that this was indeed the case. This was usually relatively easy. Most cases did differ in some respect. The exception was patients who had a condition similar to their own. They would not usually be acknowledged to have cancer unless their condition could be defined as being in some way different from the patient's own one and, therefore, not strictly comparable with it.

> Yes, they were similar to me but not exactly the same. We're all different.

> I knew some of them had cancer. But they had different treatments. They weren't exactly the same as me.

This quite highly developed awareness of other patients' conditions did not mean that cancer was talked about explicitly even among those patients who took part in discussions about their illness. On the contrary, the terms 'cancer' and 'malignancy' were very seldom used. Rather, the patients communicated by means of euphemisms where each knew what the other had but did not name the disease. This was because, although they knew what the other had, they did not know for certain whether the other knew and therefore could not risk using the term 'cancer'.

> No, we didn't speak about cancer as such. I said I was in with my throat and getting radiotherapy treatment for it. I didn't say it was cancer. It might scare them. They mightn't know that's what they had.

> We talk about it a lot and we all know what the others have got. We've all got cancer of course. But we don't say that, just vaguely. I don't think it's wise to discuss your condition with other patients. I mean, to talk about cancer. You don't know what they're thinking. You could talk about it in other ways though. We talked about it but we didn't mention that word.

It was very difficult to break out of this cycle as no patient was prepared to make the first move and introduce explicit reference to cancer and thereby risk alarming his fellow patients. Even where it became obvious that the other patient was aware that he had a malignancy, the taboo associated with the word was strong enough to prevent its use. Nor, as we shall see, was it necessary to use these explicit terms, as patients were able to communicate perfectly effectively about their illness without them. The diagnosis could be left implicit. Nevertheless, some couples or small groups did arrive at this degree of explicitness and did use these terms in their discussions but this was comparatively rare. How this degree of explicitness emerged in these groups I cannot say.

For patients who wanted to find out about their condition, of all the topics which they discussed, their illness was one of the chief ones both in terms of the time spent talking about it and of the importance to them of such conversations. But not all patients were equally active in instigating these discussions. To some extent, frequency of discussion about illness seemed to depend upon two or three individuals in the ward at any particular time who acted as catalysts for such discussion drawing into it others who would not necessarily have acted as initiators themselves but who were, nevertheless, willing participants once the discussion was under way. One of the most common times for such discussions was after the doctors had completed a ward round when patients would gather to talk about what they had said about their conditions or treatments.

What aspects of their conditions did these patients talk about? Much of the time was spent comparing notes on their progress and in interpreting events. Patients sought advice and information from each other on a variety of matters, but most questions were concerned with the interpretation of what was happening to them and the meaning of certain courses of action. Why did they get X-rays? What were the tests for? Were the doctors looking for spread of the disease? Did additional treatment mean that the disease had not been eradicated? Did getting radiotherapy instead of an operation mean that the condition was inoperable? What did the doctors mean by what they said? However, while they sought truthful answers to these questions, what in fact they received from their fellow patients was reassurance: 'They always do lots of tests in hospital. It's just routine.' 'They're probably giving you radiotherapy just to make sure.' Patients did not offer candid assessments of what they thought about another's condition. 'Let's face it, all the women in this ward have more or less the same trouble and some are worried about it. If they come up to talk about their troubles, and are worried, you try to reassure them. You don't tell them what you really think.'

We therefore had a situation where patients came together in order to obtain further information about their illness but where nobody either gave, or received, wholly truthful answers to their questions. They all wanted the truth for themselves but, at the same time, were all busy reassuring one another.

The patients also spent a lot of time comparing their experiences and progress. This was especially so if their conditions were perceived as being the same or similar (Roth 1963, pp. 16-17). Of particular concern to them was the question of why patients with apparently similar conditions should receive different forms of treatment. Did it mean that one patient's condition was worse than another's?

> Well, we do compare with each other and if somebody gets something and the other doesn't, we wonder why. A lot of patients are worried about why they get different operations or different treatment for the same thing. They think it means they're worse.

Again, in making these comparisons, the patients tried to reassure one another. To do so, they might maintain that their own condition was more serious than someone else's as the following extract demonstrates.

> Mrs Collins: Yes, but I think my condition's probably worse than yours because they didn't see fit to operate on me. I'm just getting deep rays.
> Miss Gordon: Oh, no. No, I'm quite sure that means that it wasn't bad enough to operate. I wish I'd just had what you're getting. I'm sure that, if you get an operation, it's more serious.

In seeking information and in making comparisons, patients regarded certain individuals as being potentially more fruitful sources of information than others. Those whose advice and knowledge were most sought after were the readmissions to the ward, particularly if they had started off with the same condition as the enquiring patient. They had been through the process and were, therefore, perceived as being ideally placed for providing an insight into what was likely to happen to those who were embarking upon it. By probing into the history of readmissions, patients sought to obtain some indication of what the course of their own illness might be and the likelihood that their own condition would recur. The 'veterans', however, tried to reassure them as much as possible stressing that what had happened to them would not necessarily happen to others.

A lot come to ask me for advice because I've been in here so often. 'How did you feel?' 'Was your arm sore?' 'Do you think I'll have to come back in too?' I tell them they're probably not the same as me. I seem to be giving pep talks all the time.

However, patients did not always believe other patients' reassurances any more than they accepted the doctors' ones. They would often put more faith in their observations and what they had learned about other patients' histories than in the reassurances which they received. They therefore made certain deductions which were often at variance with the optimistic interpretations which were proferred by their fellow patients. 'She had a breast off followed by radiotherapy and she's been back twice since then. I'm worried in case I follow suit. She said not to worry, that I was different, but she's just being kind.'

Clearly, those patients who sought a frank assessment of the nature of their condition were not likely to obtain it from their fellow patients. However, while the patient network operated mainly to provide reassurance, it did not succeed in convincing all patients that they need not worry about their condition. Most of them, while they derived some comfort from these encounters, retained their fears.

While the great majority of patients took great care not to cause others distress, one or two were less considerate. For example, one patient, who had been readmitted several times, told another on his first admission that his first operation would not be the end of the process and that he would be readmitted in the future. However, such instances were very rare. The predominant features of interaction on the ward were tact and reassurance.

I would like to close this chapter with a word about the atmosphere in the ward. Ward 4C was a remarkably happy one. To be sure, many of the patients were troubled but they did their best not to let this show. Interaction on the ward was therefore characterised by a cheerfulness and camaraderie which itself must have contributed to putting patients in a more equable frame of mind. The atmosphere on the ward was aptly summed up by one of the patients.

It's a very happy ward. It's surprising, isn't it, when you consider the troubles the patients have. You would expect them to be depressed but they aren't.

Notes

1. For data on the part played by relatives I had to rely upon what the patients told me they were told by them. However, given the openness with which patients usually divulged their sources of information to me, I have no reason to suspect that they obtained more information from their relatives than they were willing to reveal.
2. Not only were they often aware of what other patients had, they would also assess how bad their condition was. 'Mrs Jarvis and Mrs Williamson look like terminal cases.'
3. Defining one's own case as an exception has also been recorded among dying patients. Glaser and Strauss (1965, p. 133) note: 'Patients may deny their fate by using other patients as comparative references. Two common types of comparison are the exception and the favourable comparison. A patient using the first approach (concludes) that he is an exceptional case, that somehow the illness that caused so many others to die will not kill him: he will be cured.'

11 THE RELATIVES

In this, the penultimate chapter, I examine the ward staff's perspective on what the patients' relatives should be told and the nature and content of their communication with them. The material used here was derived from interviews with the doctors, nurses and patients and a very limited number of observations of staff-relative encounters. Relatives were not interviewed. I cannot, therefore, comment upon their awareness, desire for information or satisfaction with what was communicated to them. Nevertheless, what was clear was that, consistent with the findings of previous studies (Fitts and Ravdin 1953; Oken 1961; Quint 1964), the relatives were likely to be told much more than the patients. They would be told the truth about the patient's condition or, at least, much more of the truth than was disclosed to the patients themselves. The ward staff were all agreed that this was, and should be, the case.

However, this does not mean that information about the patient was routinely imparted to their relatives. It was not. Generally, the relatives had to take the initiative and ask for information. They would not normally be told unless they did so. Moreover, by no means all relatives enquired. A substantial proportion did not. Therefore, many relatives received no information from the hospital staff about the patient's condition. Only those who took the trouble to enquire were likely to be informed. Having said that, however, there were occasions when the doctor would seek out relatives in order to inform them about the patient. But this was limited to those instances where there was a specific reason for doing so: in particular, where the patient's condition was serious and the doctors were reasonably certain that the outlook was hopeless. In such cases, where the prognosis was clearly bad and where the patient's condition was deteriorating markedly, if they perceived that the relatives were unaware of this, the doctors might make a point of speaking to them and informing them of the gravity of the patient's condition in the belief that they should be made aware of his worsening state or forewarned and prepared for his impending demise. Nevertheless, in most cases the onus was very much on the relatives to find out about the patient. However, when they did so, unlike the patients themselves, they were likely to be put in possession of the full and genuine facts of the case.

Why was it that the doctors were prepared to tell the relatives but not the patients? This is a difficult question to answer. Certainly, the doctors themselves were often unsure of the rationale which lay behind this policy. To an extent, it was clear that it was something which had simply become recognised as the accepted practice and to which everyone adhered without questioning its basis. Therefore, the rationale behind it was not something which the doctors consciously considered or reflected upon. But, of course, when asked why this practice obtained, a number of accounts were offered: relatives had a right to be told; when the relatives asked they, unlike the patients, wanted to know the truth; someone had to make provision for the time when the patient passed away; if they had been prepared for it, the relatives would react less badly when the end came; and, if they were in possession of the full facts, they would be able to co-operate with the medical staff in the management of the patient.

> You know, I've never thought of it. I've always been brought up to think, we must tell the relatives. I think it's reflected in the fact that the relatives will then regard themselves as part of a team. They're prepared possibly to take the patient home and nurse him at home when he's obviously getting worse. Instead of standing at the doctor's door and getting in touch, 'Now, he's not getting any better, this can't go on. You've got to do something.' If they know, they'll realize that everything has been done. That there's no point in them creating, feeling that they're acting under a sense of obligation to the patient by demanding more concentrated attention and treatment in the belief that he might get better. But when they're prepared to accept these things, they're understanding. . . If they see that you've done everything you can, if a patient has been well nursed, carefully looked after, and been kept as cheery as possible, then they appreciate that and they'll play their part in visiting frequently and taking them away when you feel you can't do anything more or needing the bed, or something like that, then they'll make an extra effort to look after them when they haven't got long anyway. And, when the patient does go, then they've no sense of regret if they've realized before that everything possible has been done for the patient.

> I've often wondered this myself. But I think they all want the truth and I think they've got every right to know. It would be wrong to tell them lies. They have to cope with the patient and they have to know what's wrong with them and what they have to do.

Because there's a feeling that somebody ought to know simply because, if it's bad, there may be provisions made for children or other
. . . and in general anyway I think relatives have the moral right to
know because it's a terrible shock to them. . . I had that once or
twice in fact—patients where I didn't tell the relatives the whole truth
and then regretted not doing so afterwards because the patient died
very suddenly and the stress on the relatives was far greater than if
they'd been expecting it for quite a long time. Although it's a horrible
thing to live with, I think you should give them some idea of this. . .
severity. It's only fair on them.

There is no reason to suppose that the sentiments expressed above
did not, in fact, influence the doctors' thinking on disclosure. I would
simply suggest that, over and above these, there were probably other
compelling reasons for informing relatives. Firstly, while the staff could
to a considerable extent control the patients' information network,
given that it was confined to the ward, they could not exercise the same
measure of control over the relatives' access to information. They were
not so restricted. They had access to sources of information outside
the hospital, primarily the general practitioners, who might contradict
what they were told within it. The realization, upon receiving contradictory statements or fuller disclosure from another quarter, that
information had been withheld from them, could have provoked a
hostile and indignant reaction in relatives. In short, there was no point
in the doctors attempting to conceal information from relatives when
they could not ensure the success of such a policy and where failure
might carry the penalty of alienating them or even precipitating a clash.
Besides, while the patient would probably never know that information
had been withheld, the relatives, in many cases, ultimately and inevitably
would. They would have to be told the truth if the patient died. In that
event, of course, the doctors would then be obliged to confess that they
had previously been less than forthright. Secondly, if relatives had not
been informed of the patient's condition, his apparently sudden death
or deterioration could lead them to level accusations of incompetence
or negligence at the medical staff. Relatives who had been prepared for
these events would be much less likely to do so. Hence the doctors'
determination that, in serious cases, somebody in the patient's family
must be told. 'Then you have to tell someone in the family even if it's
the grandfather.'
  So, for a number of reasons, the doctors felt obliged to tell the relatives. But, in doing so, did they not risk something which they passion-

ately wished to avoid? The relatives might pass on the information to the patient. In practice, this threat did not materialize. Other authors had noted that collusion was likely to occur between doctors and relatives in withholding information from the patient. (Quint 1964; Glaser and Strauss 1965.) The findings in this study were no exception. As we saw in the last chapter, relatives did not communicate the diagnosis or prognosis to patients. Only if the news was good would they pass it on. The great majority of relatives shared the doctors' concern that the patient should not be told. Usually, then, it was not necessary for the doctor to attempt to persuade them to withhold information from the patient. On the contrary, it was probably more common for *the relatives* to express spontaneously to the doctors their wish that the patient should not be told.

> They don't want them to know. In most cases the relatives will say, 'I don't want her to be told.' And when you say, 'Of course, I haven't mentioned the word cancer', they say, 'Oh no. . .no, don't do that.'

> One very rarely needs to tell them not to pass it on. It's only the occasional relative who will tell the patient. So it's not really a problem. It's just pretty awful when it happens. The majority of relatives say distinctly at once that they don't want the patient told. This is very striking.

Nevertheless, there was still a risk that some relatives might be tempted to disclose and, in cases where they had not expressed the contrary view, the doctors would, as an additional insurance against this possibility, attempt to influence them. Clearly, they could not command or instruct relatives not to tell the patient. Their persuasion had to be of a more subtle kind. They would make a point of informing them that *they* were not telling the patient and suggest that, under the circumstances, it was probably to the patient's advantage that he was not told.

> Yes, but we have no real. . .no control. I mean, all you can do is suggest to them and hope they'll follow your suggestion. And usually, in the majority—well, virtually every case—this is exactly what happens. You say to them, 'Well, I think it's better he shouldn't be told . . .' and suggest that between us we thought it would be a good idea. But really it was my idea.

> We say we haven't told the patient because we feel that if we tell her

it would not do her any good. They react better to their treatment
and respond better and they've a better chance if they don't know.

However, while relatives did not deliberately convey information to
patients they might inadvertently issue certain cues to them by their
general demeanour and behaviour in their presence. The doctors were
conscious of this. But, in telling them, it was a risk which they had to
accept. For the most part, they could not control the ways in which
relatives presented themselves to patients. But, given that most of their
communication with relatives took place during the visiting hours, they
could do something to ensure that the relatives did not see the patient
while they were at their most distressed. Consequently, they tried to
see the relatives at the end of the visiting hour, after they had seen the
patient. It was hoped that they would have regained their composure
by the time of their next visit.

. . .I don't think I've ever seen a case where the relatives pass. . .
deliberately passed on bad news. But, you see, you must remember
that, if a man and woman have been living together for forty years,
there's a certain hidden rapport between them. The man knows if
the woman is telling lies. The man can look at that woman's face
and know exactly how worried she is and vice versa. So that when
we tell the relatives we tell them when they're about to leave, not
just about to see the patient. If they break down and then go in. . .
if they are suddenly confronted with this news and the mask's down
. . .they haven't enough time to consolidate their feelings and so
forth. And they break down, or they're thinking and not really
taking much notice of the patient. The patient can see through that
in a minute. So we tell the relatives when they leave rather than when
they arrive. But, even then, a lot of information gets back to the
patient. . .through the relatives. Not because they're wanting to tell
but because there's a very definite rapport between them and they
sense it.

In order to further minimise the potential cues consequent upon
their talking to relatives, the doctors might make a point of telling the
patient that they had spoken with them, describing the reasons for the
encounter in such a way as to make it appear perfectly normal and unthreatening.

Now, I'll sometimes say to a patient, 'Now your husband was on the phone, he's wanting to know just exactly what's happening to you, so I said I would see him this afternoon. . .or tomorrow.' And I'll say, 'That's fair enough, I'm pleased he rang up. It's nice of them to come and take an interest and find out from us.' Now, there again you see, you're sliding the patient off the idea: 'Oh, he's sent for him', or, 'This is a very serious talk', and we're putting the emphasis on, 'We're delighted to see the relatives—it's good that they have an interest in what we're doing', you see? Have a chat with them and they see what sort of chap I am and I like to see what sort of people they are.

While relatives were told much more than the patients, they were not all treated equally when it came to imparting information to them. It was thought appropriate to discuss the patient's condition in greater detail with some relatives than with others. By and large, the closer the relative the more they were likely to be told. 'As the relationship to the patient becomes thinner, so does the information you give out to them about the patient.' But even a close relative might not always be told. Occasionally, the doctors might feel that they could not cope with the news. Such judgements were difficult to make, being highly subjective and often based upon a single interview.

. . .it's much more difficult to tell with the relatives than it is with the patient because you see the relatives for ten minutes, not for weeks on end while they're in the ward. You talk to them once and you have to sum them up very quickly—what their reaction will be.

Nevertheless, such decisions were occasionally taken. But, given the fleeting nature of the encounters with relatives, only gross manifestations of an inability to cope with bad news would prejudice disclosure to them: '. . .unless they're obviously *extremely* neurotic or disturbed or anxious sort of people.' In cases where it was judged that the closest relative could not be told, the next in line would be informed.[1]

As with the patients, the responsibility for informing the relatives rested solely with the medical staff. But, in contrast with the accepted practice in relation to patients, *any* doctor was at liberty to inform them. Indeed, most often it was the junior doctors who saw them to discuss the patient's condition. The nursing staff, on the other hand, were expected not to disclose. Usually, though, it was the nurses who were approached by relatives in the first instance. In handling this, they followed the same drill as employed in the management of patient enquiries. They referred the relative to the doctor. They did not venture a reply to their questions. This applied to all ranks, including the Sisters.

> Staff Nurse C: I would say, 'Well, I don't know enough about it—I only nurse the patient. I'll make an appointment for you to see Dr so and so', and I do.

> Sister R: We're not supposed to tell relatives you see. We're always told to get the doctor. The nursing profession aren't supposed to reveal anything.

In fact it was usually the senior members of the nursing staff to whom relatives addressed their questions. Perhaps, as one junior nurse suggested, this was because they felt that it required someone in authority to be able to answer them. 'No, they never ask me. They kind of look at your badge and, if they see "student", they won't ask. Usually they'll ask Staff Nurse or Sister.'

However, once the relative had been put in the picture by the doctors, the nurses felt freer to respond to their queries. Certain stock replies were employed.

> They'll ask, 'How's he doing?' 'Is there any improvement?' and things like that. You say, 'No change.' Or, if terminal, 'Condition deteriorating', if obvious—only if obvious. 'She's brighter today' if there's really not much to say or, 'There's a definite improvement.'

If the nurses were not very forthcoming, what sorts of information did relatives obtain from the medical staff? Well, certainly they were told much more than the patient. However, while there was far less reluctance to tell relatives that the patient had cancer, this would not normally be volunteered to them. While relatives were informed of the diagnosis in a comparatively explicit way, the doctors would usually not use the term 'cancer' unless it had first been introduced by the relatives themselves. Instead, the relatives would be told that the patient had a 'tumour' or 'growth' or, even, a 'malignant growth'. The doctors varied in the terms which they preferred to use.

Before the condition had been confirmed as malignant, relatives would be alerted to the possibility that it could be something serious. 'I'm a bit worried about this. I think there might be something serious there. But we're going to find out.'

Thereafter they would be informed of the diagnosis. However, the degree of explicitness with which this was done varied according to the perceived severity of the patient's condition. Only in cases where the possibility of a cure was assessed to be remote would the relative be informed that the disease was cancer.

> I use the word 'malignant growth' and they accept that. But I wouldn't have the same hesitation in using the word 'cancer' to the relatives. In a hopeless case, that is. I wouldn't use it in an operable case.

In more hopeful cases, telling them that the condition was 'malignant' was as far as the doctors were prepared to go. While rendering this diagnosis, they would emphasise that the outlook was good. 'Well, it is malignant and it's got to be dealt with. But we haven't found any evidence of spread or anything and we think she should be OK.'

But why were they unwilling to go the whole way and tell the relatives explicitly what the patient had? The reason seemed to be that 'cancer' was believed to be an excessively emotive word and the doctors felt that there was no point in alarming relatives unduly by mentioning it, if the outlook was favourable. Only if relatives asked directly would they be told that the patient had cancer. Then they would always be told the truth. Again, though, this disclosure would be accompanied by a statement to the effect that they believed that it could be cured. 'They may ask if it's cancer. You say to them, "Yes, I'm afraid it is." "But", you add, "there's no evidence of spread and I'm hoping everything will be all right."'

Compared with the patients, relatives were both more likely to ask questions and more pointed in their questioning when they did enquire. It was not unusual for them to ask if the patient had cancer. We have seen that such a direct enquiry evoked an equally frank response. Nor did they hesitate to enquire about the prognosis: 'How bad is it?' 'Has it spread?' 'Will it come back after it's treated?' 'Will this be a cure?' or even, 'How long has he got to live?' How much success did they have in finding out about these matters?

In response to questions relating to the prognosis, relatives were told the truth. If the prognosis was good, it presented no problem. The relatives were told that the outlook was hopeful.

> Well, it's a malignant growth but we're treating it in the usual way and we expect everything to be all right. As far as we know, it hasn't spread and the outlook should be good.

> I'm afraid, as you know, she had a cancer of the breast. But we've

operated on it and the prospects are good. She has a good chance of being cured so you shouldn't worry.

But, even if the prognosis was bad, the relatives, upon enquiring, would be told that this was the case. However, the rendering of such a frank assessment of the projected course and outcome for the patient's condition was always accompanied by an expression of optimism. Relatives were not divested of all hope. A degree of hope was often conveyed by stressing that the patient would continue to be treated and that, therefore, by implication, the doctors had not entirely abandoned all hope of a cure. The extent to which optimism was expressed depended upon the severity of the patient's condition.

Husband, wife, son, daughter or father or mother; they would be told everything. They'd be told your problems: that the disease has spread and there's little we can do but we'll try. Even then, you've got to leave them some glimmer of hope, however faint it is. In that . . . 'Of course there are cases of cancer that disappear quite spontaneously without any sort of treatment whatsoever and this might be one of them, we can't say. I don't think it is, but it could be and we've just got to work on from day to day.'

If they ask if it has spread, generally you would say 'Yes'. But you shouldn't remove all their hope. You can tell them it's spread but that you're treating it and you're hoping it will work although you can't say for sure that it will.

In some cases, though, where the patient's death was regarded as inevitable and imminent, it was not possible to profess optimism. Under those circumstances, the relative would be told, as gently as possible, that the outlook was hopeless.

'We can't really do much more for your father. This treatment's only palliative. It's really only a matter of time before the disease overcomes him.'

If the relative says, 'She's going to die isn't she?' or something like that, then you would say, 'Well, I'm afraid she is, yes.' Providing, of course, you were sure that the case was hopeless yourself.

Occasionally, the fact that the outlook was hopeless would be volunteered to the relatives. However, an unqualified bad prognosis would not be volunteered to them unless it was felt that the illness had reached a stage at which it was necessary that they should be made aware of its grave nature. What the relatives would seldom be given was an estimated *time* of death. Unless, of course, the patient was in the terminal stages of the illness and it was confidently expected that he would die within the following day or two. 'I never give them a specific time. We're very vague about that. Unless the patient's actually terminal and dying when I say, "Well, maybe forty eight hours or so."'

The doctors' reluctance to predict a time of death was due to the fact that they quite simply were usually unable to do so with any accuracy.

> Well, you know, people have seen too many films where the relatives wander in and the doctor says, 'He's got six months.' Or 'He's got eighteen months left.' And the patient lives for nineteen months and they think he's been cured. Well this is just nonsense. Nobody knows how long a patient. . .you've got a fair idea in many cases, but in the vast majority of cases you've no idea. Sometimes you can't even say weeks rather than months or years. I suppose really—and this is how we tackle it—we try to get over to the relative that it might be a matter of weeks or months.

In addition, of course, a premature proclamation of imminent death could lead to considerable embarrassment if not fulfilled (Sudnow 1967, pp. 93-94). Questions about how long the patient had to live therefore received rather vague replies. 'Well, you can never tell with their condition. It could be weeks or it could be a couple of months.'

Apart from the doctors' reluctance to predict the time of death, clearly relatives were well informed about the patient's condition. Certainly, they were told much more than the patients themselves. Several suggestions were advanced for why this should be so. However, the extent to which they were kept informed depended upon whether or not they enquired. Those relatives who did not do so were not likely to be told unless it was felt that the patient's condition was sufficiently grave to warrant seeking them out.

Note

1. This concurs with Glaser and Strauss's finding (1965, p. 145) that, 'The general procedure is to disclose first to the closest or most intimate family member deemed strong enough to take the blow.'

12 SUMMARY AND CONCLUSION

The purpose of this book has been to describe and explain the structure and organization of the processes of communication associated with malignant disease in one particular hospital context. Unlike the bulk of previous work on communication with cancer sufferers, the present study dealt with patients with diagnosed but undisclosed malignancy. A further point of departure from previous approaches to the subject was a concern with the processual and interactional nature of the phenomena to be investigated. A central feature of this approach was an examination of the ways in which processes of communication and patterns of adaptation evolved and developed over the course of patients' hospitalization in response to changing contexts and the actions of the participants to extend or control awareness and to manage the flow of information. As such, it was in the tradition of previous work on tuberculosis (Roth, 1963), polio (Davis, 1963), and the dying (Glaser and Strauss 1965). The primary focus was upon how the various participants coped with uncertainty.

The cornerstone of the doctors' philosophy on telling was the belief that the great majority of patients should not be told. This was based upon assumptions about patients' desire for information and their probable reaction to disclosure. They assumed that patients did not want to know and would react badly if they were told. Their overriding concern was to leave the patient with hope. At the same time, though, they acknowledged that some patients would genuinely want to know and expressed the view that, where such patients could be counted upon not to react unfavourably, they should be informed. However, the translation of this ideological position into action was not a straightforward matter. Its implementation had to take account of a number of attendant uncertainties. Uncertainty was endemic to the treatment of cancer patients. The doctors experienced considerable uncertainty over strictly clinical matters. At certain stages, they could often not be certain of the diagnosis and prognosis. In addition, there was also a great deal of uncertainty associated with what to communicate to patients. The doctors could not be sure of how much patients wanted to know or how they were likely to react to disclosure. This latter type of uncertainty accompanied every case. There was, therefore, no certain basis on which to make decisions about whether or not to tell particular patients. In response to this, the doctors adopted a policy of not disclosing to any patient unless it was absolutely necessary.

Uncertainty was then a central factor in determining the nature and extent of communication to patients about their illness. However, the doctors were not explicitly conscious of problems of uncertainty in the course of their everyday work. They were not constantly grappling with the question of what to tell patients or with uncertainty about whether patients wanted to know and how they would react if they were told. This was because all communication to patients was routinized. The routine ways of handling these potential problems ensured that they seldom surfaced as explicit or conscious problematic issues. These routine procedures were grounded in the doctors' philosophy and constituted ways of implementing it in situations of uncertainty. In other words, they provided the doctors with ways of managing uncertainty consistent with their beliefs about patients' desire for information and probable reactions to disclosure.

The routines were geared to limiting the amount of disclosure to patients. There were routine procedures pertaining to what was volunteered to patients and a separate set of routine responses to specific types of patient demand. These routines were differentially appropriate for different categories of condition, in terms of severity, at different stages of their treatment. That is, telling was based upon typifications of cases. A central feature of these routines was the way in which professions of certainty or uncertainty were used in the management of communication and to limit the degree of disclosure to patients. These routine procedures had evolved over time. They were admirably adapted to accommodating and coping with the many problems which the doctors potentially faced in communicating with the patients. They covered almost every contingency. The only occasions on which the doctor might disclose were if the patient persistently demanded the truth or if he refused treatment. The routinization of communication ensured consistency in what patients were told and obviated the necessity of making decisions in individual cases. The doctors simply implemented the routines appropriate to particular types of case. All the doctors employed the same routine ways of communicating with the patients. While the detail of what patients in the same category were told could differ, the substance remained constant. Had it not been accomplished in a routine manner, it is almost certain that, given the irresolvable nature of the uncertainties associated with it, the task of communicating with cancer patients would have been fraught with a great many more difficulties. These, then, were the methods of communication and devices for controlling information employed by the ward staff. How did the patients manage *their* uncertainty in that context?

On admission to the ward, the overwhelming majority of patients knew or suspected that they had a malignancy. Most of them only suspected and few of them had much idea of their prognosis. They were, therefore, subject to a great deal of uncertainty about the nature and severity of their illness. However, they handled their suspicions, and the uncertainty consequent upon them, in very different ways. It was hypothesized that patients would attempt to cope with uncertainty by seeking information about their condition. This was found to be so. But there were crucial differences in the sort of information which patients sought and in where they sought it. Only a minority of patients sought to eradicate their uncertainty by trying to find out *the truth* about their condition. The hypothesis that patients would attempt to manage their uncertainty by seeking the truth presupposed that they would want to know. Many of them did not. Almost 70 per cent of those who suspected did not want confirmation of their diagnosis. Even fewer wanted information on their prognosis. They preferred uncertainty to knowing because it was precisely that uncertainty which afforded them hope. Thus, it was only those patients who wanted to know who proceeded by seeking to establish the truth. But, those patients who did not want to know also tried to manage uncertainty by seeking information. However, it was information seeking of a different nature. They sought exclusively information which would reinforce an optimistic conception of their condition. They tried to confirm that they might not have cancer or that the outlook was good. A purely passive rejection of the possible diagnosis and prognosis was not enough. Those patients could not simply deny the possibility that they might have cancer or that the outlook might be bad. They had to continually work at it by seizing upon and interpreting appropriately those cues which could sustain a hopeful conception, and by rationalizing or otherwise negating the importance of those which might suggest the contrary. Such information seeking and distillation was confined to the informal contexts as they offered the patients a greater measure of control over the acquisition and interpretation of information.

Now it might be argued that, had the patients been in a context where a more liberal approach to telling obtained, more of them would have expressed a desire to find out about their illness. In other words, the argument goes, the patients in the present study might have been inhibited from enquiring about their condition by their perception that the doctors did not want to tell them, the corollary of this being that,

had they been in a setting where they believed that information would
be made readily available to them, they would have been more likely to
both express a desire to know and to enquire. That is, a different context, in terms of orientations towards telling, could have structured patients' expressed desires for information and their consequent actions in
a very different way. However, I consider this to be unlikely for two
reasons. Firstly, patients who did not want to know indicated their preference upon admission to the ward and before they had been able to
gauge the sort of orientation which obtained there. Secondly, and more
importantly perhaps, while they accepted that their diagnosis and prognosis would probably not be volunteered to them, they nearly all anticipated that they would be told if they asked. In other words, *they* did
not know that the doctors would not tell them nor did they perceive
the context as being a restrictive one.

Whether or not patients sought to eradicate uncertainty by seeking
the truth was found to be a product of their perception of cancer in
general and their assessment of the severity of their own condition in
particular. It was those patients for whom the truth about their condition would not destroy their hope completely who sought to eliminate
uncertainty in this way.[1] But finding out the truth about their condition
was not easy. As we saw, the practices of communication employed by
the ward staff were specifically designed to prevent such disclosure. This
meant, of course, that their diagnosis and prognosis were not volunteered
to them, the routines also made it very difficult for them to obtain the
information they wanted by asking. In a sense, the routine procedures
were a product of the actions of the patient group itself. One of the
more fundamental assumptions underlying the doctors' policy was that
the patients did not want to know. This was justified by pointing to the
fact that few of them asked. Thus, the routines were both a product of,
and sustained by, the actions of the patient group as a whole and the
doctors' consequent perception of their wishes. This was ideal for the
majority of patients who did not want to know. But, being tailored to
meet the perceived wishes of the majority, these routines were detrimental to the fulfilment of the wishes of the minority, making it
extremely difficult for them to find out what they wanted to know.[2]

But patients who wanted to find out the truth about their condition
were not entirely frustrated by not being able to obtain it formally.
They were often able to find out what they wanted to know in other
ways.[3] In fact, what they were told by the doctors often contained all
they wanted to know. Many deduced that they had cancer from what
was communicated to them by identifying what they were told as being

euphemistic and interpreting it accordingly. Whether the doctor 'told' or not depended on the patient's desire to know the truth. Patients who were 'told' in this way were self-selective in that only those who wanted to know would interpret what they were told as meaning that they had cancer. At the same time, what was communicated to the patients was sufficiently ambiguous to enable those who did not want to know to maintain the belief that they might not have the disease. In addition, of course, patients were able to obtain indications of the nature and severity of their condition from a number of cues or informal sources of information. They would also frequently discuss their illness with each other and compare notes. However, such discussions were characterized by mutual reassurance and the avoidance of explicit reference to the disease. Those who sought a frank assessment of the nature of their condition were not likely to obtain it from their fellow patients.

While a good many patients did not need to ask or were able to obtain the information they sought in other ways, for many others, who sought to confirm their suspicions through direct enquiry, the truth remained elusive. However, it is difficult to be critical of the staff for not responding to questions with full disclosure. Some of their assumptions were justified. A great many patients did not want to know. Moreover, they could not be sure of the status of patient questioning. However, contrary to what they assumed, those who asked directly did want to know. Patients who asked about their condition wanted to know precisely what they asked. In chapter 8 I discussed the problems involved in generalizing this finding to other contexts. This applied in particular to relatively inexplicit questions like 'What is it?' which could be asked by any patient, whether they suspected cancer or not. However, if the reply to such a question did not in itself confirm their suspicions, those patients would often go on to ask the more explicit questions: 'Is it cancer?' or 'Is it malignant?'. Patients who posed those direct questions very definitely did want to know and were prepared to accept a positive answer. This is probably true for all patients who ask so directly given the unequivocal and irrevocable nature of the enquiries.

The findings summarised in the preceding pages could only have been obtained by means of a combination of research methods. Interviews were essential for obtaining certain sorts of information. Similarly, examination of the processual nature of the topic of investigation, and detailed information on what the participants did, could not have been achieved without observation. The data yielded through observation also illustrated an important theoretical-methodological point: peoples' perceptions or accounts of what they do and their actual practices may differ considerably. This was demonstrated in a particularly striking way in relation to the doctors' practices of telling. When asked about their communication practices the doctors maintained that they depended upon their perception and assessment of the individual case. Clearly, this account was not borne out by observation of what they actually did. Communication was routinized. Based solely upon their own accounts, a summary of the doctors' practices of communication would have looked radically different. It would have stressed the importance of decision making in individual cases. Such an account would have been considerably at variance with what actually happened. This finding could not have been obtained through interviewing alone and it questions further the validity and usefulness of the interview as a device for the study of social processes or for establishing what people do.

The combination of observation and interviewing was well-suited to the task at hand. Certainly one can have reasonable confidence in those data concerned with description of what occurred. However, those pertaining to questions of motivation, or why people behaved as they did, are a different matter. Here certain aspects of the problem remained hidden, approximate or not subject to ultimate verification. While there was no reason to doubt the causal significance of the explanations for their actions advanced by both doctors and patients, it was not possible to establish their underlying motivations with certainty. This may be partly a purely technical problem. No matter how sensitive one's research instruments, it is not possible to establish conclusively what people 'really' think or what their 'real' reasons for action are. Short of looking inside people's heads, we must ultimately rely upon what they tell us they think. However, it is not simply the fact that people may lie or deliberately conceal their underlying motivations which renders such accounts problematic. Even if it were possible to look inside heads, or to develop our research instruments to such a degree that it was possible to uncover peoples' 'real' motivations, it is doubtful if we would find consistent, discrete and immutable underlying reasons for action. Such an attempt would presuppose that people do have 'real' reasons or cohesive sets of motivations which inform what they do. It is questionable whether such 'real' motivations exist. Rather, individuals' motivations are probably so infinitely complex that they are often imperfectly understood even by the individuals themselves. It is interesting that patients were often unclear as to why they did or did not want to know. The reasons were probably complex, difficult to reflect upon, and operated at the level of a feeling state rather than as a conscious cognitive process and, therefore, were extremely difficult, if not impossible, to articulate. In this sort of situation, the explanation which is offered is likely to be only one of several possible ones each of which probably has some claim to the status of a reason for action. In short, it is likely that action is a product of a multiplicity of ideas, desires and attitudes the relative import of which may not be fully understood even by the subject himself. Any search for 'real' reasons is likely, therefore, to become marooned in a quagmire of non-assessable, and sometimes conflicting, motivations.

A search for motivation is occasioned by the belief that people have sets of attitudes and desires on which they base their actions and that, furthermore, these motivations can be identified. Clearly people do not act in a cognitive and ideational void, but the above paradigm may assume an over-rational model of social action. People may only rarely have consciously thought out plans of action. Rather, they may have a vague notion of what they wish to do and simply respond, in accordance with it, to the specific inputs which they receive from the contexts in which they find themselves. However, insofar as they do have plans of action, whatever intentions an individual has will be mediated by the context in which they seek expression. In other words, actions are probably also context dependent. It is doubtful to what extent people can have a carefully worked out plan of action which they can pursue without diversion. They will be subject to the actions of others and changing events and circumstances. Such planned courses of action may, therefore, have to be modified or adapted to the requirements and constraints of particular contexts. This clearly obtained in the present study. In communication with each other both parties, that is, doctor and patient, were subject to constraints imposed by the context of the interaction itself. For example, the doctors were unable to implement their declared intention of informing selected patients. It is also interesting that relatively few of those patients who wanted their diagnosis asked directly if they had cancer. Whether they did so or not could well have been partly dependent upon the nature and context of their interactions with the doctors. It was one thing to make up one's mind to ask that question and quite another, given the implications of the possible reply and the taboo nature of the word 'cancer', to carry such a decision into practice. However much a patient might have intended asking that question, he may have found either that the opportunity for doing so did not arise or that it seemed somehow inappropriate in the context of the specific encounter. Instead he might simply ask, 'What is it?' An additional and related constraint was the fact that the doctor introduced the level at which communication should be conducted and it might have been very difficult for the patient to breach this norm.

Action is, therefore, probably, only partly rationalistic or consciously worked out in advance. Any planned course of action is likely to be modified or subverted by the constraints imposed by the context in which it is to be implemented. As such, action is likely to be a product of an interactive process between the action decided upon and the exigencies and practicalities of particular situations.

The status of the data on motivation and its relation to action is probably impossible to establish conclusively. But, while there are problems associated with the status and interpretation of interview data, we are not entirely helpless in attempting to assess the validity of such information. To an extent, the material obtained in interview could be checked by observing what the subjects did. In this way it was possible to relate peoples' accounts to what they actually did by observing how they were, or were not, translated into action. In the present study it was found that, apart from the doctors' assertion that telling was based upon the assessment of individual cases, accounts and behaviour matched. Subject to the constraints of the contexts in which they were expressed, the actions of both doctors and patients were consistent with their declared intentions and their preferred rationales for action. For example, those patients who said they wanted to know did, without exception, seek to find out the truth about their illness while those who said they preferred not to know made no attempt to do so. Thus, despite the acknowledged limitations of interview data, consistency in subjects' accounts over time, and the apparent logical expression of these attitudes in their observed behaviour, would suggest at least a tentative causal connection between the two. Nevertheless, certain problems still remain. Even then, one cannot unreservedly ascribe direct causal significance to subjects' accounts of their motives. Consistency between account and behaviour does not constitute proof of a causal relationship. Indeed, consistency would be expected whether the account accurately reflected the underlying motivation for action or not. It is, after all, in the nature of an account that, in order to be acceptable, it must be demonstrably plausible in all respects. It is quite possible, therefore, that motives other than those offered in accounts could provide the basis for action. However, no alternative explanations for the subjects' actions emerged over the course of the present investigation. In view of this, the fact that the subjects' declared intentions and the reasons which they advanced for them were plausible, consistent and in accord with the observable events to which they related would suggest that we can conclude with some justification, that the actions of the doctors and patients were probably in large part, if not wholly, a product of the reasons which they themselves advanced. There was no reason to believe otherwise.

Clearly, this study is not a definitive analysis of communication associated with cancer. Much work remains to be done on the topic. The present study itself gives rise to suggestions for further research of both sociological and clinical interest. Clearly, in view of some of the findings in this study, it is important to examine the processes of communication and their implications, in settings where, the policy of the doctors is to tell patients what they have. A comparative study of communication on general surgical wards where cues and, hence, patients' awareness might not be so pronounced would also be useful. This study was confined to the hospital context. We know relatively little about the problems, methods of communication, and processes of adaptation in the community. Accordingly, further study could focus upon the role of the general practitioner in the total communication process and the problems which he faces in managing communication with cancer patients. Similarly, of course, the question of what happens after patients are discharged from hospital is an important one. Very different patterns of adaptation may become manifest once patients are in the environment of their own homes and research on discharged cancer patients is strongly indicated. More extensive work is also required on relatives of cancer patients. For example, how aware are they, how much do they want to know, how do they cope with uncertainty, what problems do they face in interacting with the patients and how do they handle them? Finally, studies of the management of uncertainty in other settings would be of value both for comparative purposes and for enhancing our understanding of the ways in which it was managed in the present context.

This has been a tale of hope: the doctors' overriding concern to leave patients with hope; the desperate need of most patients to retain some semblance of hope; the clinging to hope despite evidence to the contrary; and the desperate search for signs of hope where, very often, little existed. There will always be anxiety associated with cancer, whether it is grounded in uncertainty or in patients' knowledge of their condition. It is not possible on the basis of this study to say which is the greater source of stress. However, what the study did reveal was that a great many patients chose for themselves the anxiety resulting from uncertainty. In this they were aided by the methods of communication employed by the staff. The fact that they were not told explicitly enabled many patients to retain hope and to construct, out of the cues available to them, a hopeful conception of their condition for themselves. Apart from enabling them to retain hope, this method of communication had the additional merit of allowing the patient to decide how much he wanted to know and of putting the onus on him to initiate a more explicit form of communication with the doctors if he so desired. He could retain the euphemistic form of communication introduced by the staff or he could move it, in varying degrees, to a more explicit form. Of course, as we saw, achievement of the latter was not easy. Because the doctors could never be certain if the patient 'really' wanted to know even if he asked outright, responses to enquiries tended to be hedged in euphemisms and evasion. Nevertheless, the doctors' communication practices, together with informal sources of information, did, to some extent, enable the patient to regulate the communication process and his receipt of information in accordance with his own needs or wishes, allowing him to find out as much, or as little, as he wanted to know.

Much has been written about the doctor's duty to divulge, fully and frankly, the nature of his condition to the patient. However, it would appear that a conservative policy on telling (that is, not volunteering the diagnosis and prognosis to patients) has much to recommend it. I would submit that it is as unwarranted to tell a patient who might not want to know as it is not to tell a patient who does want to know. The evidence of this study suggests that many patients might not want to know. However, a conservative policy on telling has other implications, particularly for public education about cancer and lay conceptions of the disease. The fact that patients are not told, even if they have a curable cancer, helps to perpetuate the lay belief that it is a dread and incurable disease. The public seldom hear of people who have been cured because, to such patients, the nature of the disease is rarely made explicit. However, when a patient dies the diagnosis is no longer a secret. Therefore, it tends to be only the more serious or fatal examples of the disease that come to the public's attention. Telling patients that they had cancer, particularly those with the more curable forms of the disease, could help to redress the balance somewhat and might serve to remove some of the mystique and dread from the public's conception of the illness. However, while well aware of this problem, the doctors in the study did not feel that they could attempt to solve it by adopting a more forthright policy on telling. To have done so in the present climate of lay opinion about the disease would, they felt, no matter how much they disclaimed its severity, simply have greatly alarmed the patients. In a sense, then, it was those very lay beliefs themselves which prevented attempts being made to remove them in the hospital context. Public education about the disease was regarded as a prerequisite for any change in hospital policy.

I have sought in these pages to present a dispassionate analysis of the processes of communication in the ward under study. No criticism of the doctors' practices is intended, and I would hope that none is implied, in the foregoing text. After all, although the study revealed that those patients who enquired did genuinely want to know, the doctors engaged in their treatment had, at that time, no way of gauging accurately the status of patient questioning. All the staff involved in caring for these patients impressed me with the sincerity of their beliefs and their overriding concern for the welfare, both physical and mental, of the patients in their care. Certainly, the staffs' concern and attention was greatly appreciated by the patients themselves. The great majority of them spontaneously expressed how delighted and grateful they were for the care which they received and were loud in their praise of the medical and nursing staff. If the doctors' communication practices can be faulted the fault is likely to be the product of a very genuine concern for their patients' wellbeing.

The problems which doctors face in communicating with cancer patients are not subject to easy solution. Even if it were possible to erect a blueprint which would indicate what each and every patient should be told, its utility would be questionable. To quote Glaser and Strauss, 'criteria that require "intimate knowledge of each patient" offer no better a solution to the doctor's dilemma than does a universally applied rule of telling or not telling' (Glaser and Strauss, 1965, p. 135). However, any 'universally applied' policy is bound to have limitations in terms of satisfying the needs of each individual and in dealing successfully with all exigencies. While, by the nature of their orientation, the practices of communication observed on Ward 4C did not fully meet the needs of all patients, they did, together with the informal sources of information, probably come fairly close to that ideal. However, basically 'conservative' policies can, of course, differ in the degree to which they enable patients who want to know to find out about their condition. This study suggests that patients who ask for their diagnosis or enquire about the extent of their illness do want to know and should therefore probably be informed. Had those patients who enquired received the information they sought more readily, the needs of nearly all the patients would have been met in full. Apart from that modification, given the practical impossibility of determining with any certainty what individual patients should and could be told,[4] there is only one real alternative to a conservative policy: namely, one of routinely informing all patients. Such a policy might not only, at least initially, cause considerable distress to many but, were patients who enquire directly to receive the information which they request, it would also be largely unnecessary. It could, of course, always be argued that, despite patients saying that they did not want to know, they would nevertheless be happier and would adjust better to their illness if they were told. All I can say in response to that is that, on the basis of my findings, this is not what many patients themselves anticipated. The policy which this study indicates is, then, one which, while not endorsing the volunteering of their diagnosis or prognosis to patients, is, at the same time, sufficiently flexible to enable those patients who ask explicitly, to be able to obtain the information which they seek in clear and unambiguous terms at the first time of asking. However, my main objective in this study was not to critically assess practices of communication: to validate or reject them. My purpose has simply been to attempt to describe and explain the processes of communication associated with malignant disease in one particular setting and to tell it as it was.

Notes

1. This discussion gives clues to the ways in which people may manage uncertainty in other contexts. Normally individuals will attempt to relieve uncertainty by seeking information. At best it induces discomfort while at worst it is productive of fear. However, if, as in the case of some cancer patients, the anxiety consequent upon knowledge is assessed as being likely to exceed that grounded in uncertainty, people will not necessarily respond to it by seeking information. If we generalize this finding to other situations we can deduce some general principles on how people may manage uncertainty. If alternatives are equally pleasant or unthreatening, or if they judge one alternative, the desired one, to be more likely than another, people will seek to eliminate uncertainty by seeking information. If, however, of the alternatives, the least desired is thought to be the more likely, people may not so readily seek to eliminate uncertainty, preferring instead to retain the hope that the more desired alternative will occur.
2. Not only was it difficult for patients to find out the truth, they would often in response to their enquiries, receive a more hopeful account of their condition than could be justified by the evidence at hand. In consequence, patients who came to an awareness of their diagnosis or prognosis on their own, through the interpretation of cues or what they were told, often had a more accurate picture of their condition than those who tried to find out by asking.
3. Of course, the fact that patients were able to find out what they wanted to know in other ways meant that their desire for information was only partly reflected in the numbers who enquired formally, thereby adding weight to the assumption that the overwhelming majority did not want to know.
4. Despite the assertion of many doctors that each case should be treated on its merits, it would appear that in practice the vast majority opt either for a policy

of telling nearly all their patients or one of usually not disclosing to anyone (Glaser and Strauss 1965; Fitts and Ravdin 1953; Oken 1961). The main advantage of these policies lies precisely in the fact that, given the uncertain nature of such judgements, they avoid the making of decisions in individual cases.

TABLES

Table 1 Patients' Awareness and Desire for Information

Group	No. of patients	Awareness	Want Diagnosis	Want Prognosis
1	32	Suspected	No	No
2	9	Suspected	Yes	No
3	14	Knew	—	No
4	6	Suspected	Yes	Yes
5	3	Knew	—	Yes
6	1	Knew	—	—
7	6	Did not suspect		
8	3	Misled into believing that they did not have cancer		
9	6	Benign—diagnosis and prognosis unproblematic		

Table 2 Desire for Confirmation of their Diagnosis among Patients who Suspected that they had Cancer

	Wanted confirmation	Did not want confirmation	Total
No.	15	32	47
%	32	68	100

BIBLIOGRAPHY

Aitken-Swan, J. and Easson, E.C. (1959):
   'Reactions of cancer patients on being told their diagnosis' *British Medical Journal*, 1, pp. 779-783.
Becker, H.S. and Geer, B. (1957):
   'Participant Observation and Interviewing: A Comparison' *Human Organisation*, 16, No. 3, pp. 28-32.
Cartwright, A. (1964):
   Human Relations and Hospital Care Routledge and Kegan Paul.
Caudill, W. (1958):
   The Psychiatric Hospital as a Small Society Harvard University Press.
Cicourel, A.V. (1964):
   Method and Measurement in Sociology Free Press.
Coser, R.L. (1962):
   Life in the Ward Michigan State University Press.
Davis, F. (1963):
   Passage Through Crisis Bobbs-Merrill.
Davis, F. (1966):
   'Uncertainty in Medical Prognosis, Clinical and Functional' In Scott, W.R. and Volkart, E.H. (ed) *Medical Care,* pp. 311-321, Wiley, New York.
Denzin, N.K. (1970):
   The Research Act in Sociology. A Theoretical Introduction to Sociological Methods. London, Butterworths.
Fitts, W.T. and Ravdin, I.S. (1953):
   'What Philadelphia physicians tell patients with cancer' *Journal of the American Medical Association,* pp. 153, 901.
Freidson, E. (1970):
   Professional Dominance: The Social Structure of Medical Care Atherton, New York.
Freidson, E. (1961):
   Patients' Views of Medical Practice Russell Sage Foundation, New York.
Gerle, B. et al (1960):
   'The patient with inoperable cancer from the psychiatric and social standpoints' *Cancer,* 13, p. 1206.
Gilbertson, V.A. and Wangensteen, O.H. (1962):

'Should the doctor tell the patient that the disease is cancer?' *Cancer*, 12, p. 82.

Glaser, B.G. and Strauss, A.L. (1965):
   Awareness of Dying Chicago, Aldine Publishing Company.

Glaser, B.G. and Strauss, A.L. (1967):
   The Discovery of Grounded Theory: Strategies for Qualitative Research London, Weidenfeld and Nicholson.

Glaser, B.G. and Strauss, A.L. (1964):
   'Awareness Contexts and Social Interaction *American Sociological Review,* Vol. 29, No. 5, pp. 669-78.

Glaser, B.G. and Strauss, A.L. (1965):
   'Temporal Aspects of Dying as a Non-Scheduled Status Passage' *American Journal of Sociology,* 71, pp. 48-59.

Gold, R.L. (1958):
   'Roles in Sociological Field Observations' *Social Forces,* 36, pp. 217-223.

Goode, W.J. and Hatt, P.K. (1952):
   Methods in Social Research McGraw-Hill.

Harris, R.J.C. (ed) (1970):
   What we Know About Cancer Allen and Unwin.

Hinton, J. (1967):
   Dying Pelican.

Kelly, W.D. and Friesen, S.R. (1950):
   'Do Cancer Patients Want To Be Told?' *Surgery,* 27 p. 822.

Kubler-Ross, E. (1969):
   On Death and Dying New York, The Macmillan Company.

McCall, G.J. and Simmons, J.L. (1969):
   Issues in Participant Observation: A Text and Reader Addison-Wesley Publishing Co.

McIntosh, J. (1974):
   'Processes of Communication, Information Seeking and Control Associated with Cancer: A Selective Review of the Literature' *Social Science and Medicine,* Vol. 8, pp. 167-187.

McIntosh, J. (1976):
   'Patients' Awareness And Desire For Information About Diagnosed But Undisclosed Malignant Disease' *Lancet,* Vol. II, p. 300.

Oken, D. (1961):
   'What To Tell Cancer Patients' *Journal of the American Medical Association,* Vol. 175, pp. 1120-1128.

Paterson, R. and Aitken-Swan, J. (1954):
   'Public Opinion on Cancer' *Lancet,* October 23, p. 857.

Quint, J.C. (1965):
'Institutionalised Practices of Information Control' *Psychiatry,* 28, pp. 119-132.

Quint, J.C. (1964):
'Mastectomy—Symbol of Cure or Warning Sign?' *GP,* Vol. 29, pp. 119-124.

Robinson, W.S. (1969):
'The Logical Structure of Analytic Induction' in McCall, G.J. and Simmons, J.L. *Issues in Participant Observation* Addison-Wesley, 196-205.

Roth, J.A. (1963):
Timetables Bobbs Merrill.

Roth, J.A. (1958):
'Ritual and Magic in the Control of Contagion' In Jaco, E.G. (ed) *Patients, Physicians and Illness* New York, Free Press, pp. 229-234.

Roth, J.A. (1963):
'Information and the Control of Treatment in Tuberculosis Hospitals' in Freidson, E. (ed) *The Hospital in Modern Society* pp. 293-318, New York, Free Press.

Rothenberg, A. (1961):
'Psychological Problems in Terminal Cancer Management' *Cancer* 14, p. 1063.

Scheff, T.J. (1963):
'Decision rules, types of error, and their consequences in medical diagnosis' *Behavioural Science,* 8 pp. 97-107.

Scheff, T.J. (1968):
'Typification in Rehabilitation Agencies' In Rubington, E. and Weinberg, M.S. *Deviance: the Interactionist Perspective* pp. 120-124. Macmillan.

Scott, M.B. and Lyman, S.M. (1970):
'Accounts, Deviance and Social Order' in J.D. Douglas (ed) *Deviance and Respectability: The Social Construction of Moral Meanings* Basic Books, pp. 89-119.

Shands, H.C. et al (1951):
'Psychological mechanisms in patients with cancer' *Cancer* 4, pp. 1159-1170.

Skipper, J.K. (1965):
'Communication and the hospitalised patient' in Skipper, J.K. and Leonard, R.C. (eds) *Social Interaction and Patient Care* J.B. Lippincott, Philadelphia pp. 61-82.

Stacey, M. (1969):
   Methods of Social Research Pergamon Press.
Standard, S. and Nathan, H. (1965):
   Should the Patient Know the Truth? New York, Springer Publishing
   Co. Inc.
Stanton, A.H. and Schwartz, M.S. (1954):
   The Mental Hospital Basic Books, New York.
Strauss, A.L. et al (1964):
   Psychiatric Ideologies and Institutions Free Press.
Sudnow, D. (1967):
   Passing on: The Social Organisation of Dying New York, Prentice-
   Hall.
Sudnow, D. (1968):
   'Normal Crimes' In Rubington, E. and Weinberg, M.S. *Deviance: The
   Interactionist Perspective* pp. 158-169, Macmillan.
Verwoerdt, A. (1966):
   Communication with the fatally ill Charles C. Thomas, Springfield,
   Illinois.
Wakefield, J. (1970):
   'The social Context of Cancer' In R.J.C. Harris (ed) *What We Know
   About Cancer* Allen and Unwin, London pp. 211-232.

INDEX